THE DANCING SPANIARDS

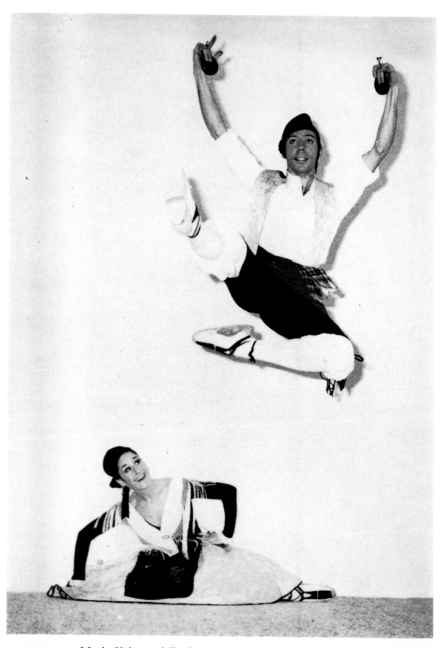

Maria Vejer and Enrique Burgos in ' Jota Aragonesa '.

THE DANCING SPANIARDS

➤·•))))◉◉◉⦿⦿⦿(((·◄

ANNA IVANOVA

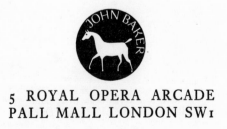

5 ROYAL OPERA ARCADE
PALL MALL LONDON SW1

First published in 1970 by
JOHN BAKER (PUBLISHERS) LTD
5 Royal Opera Arcade
Pall Mall, London SW1

SBN 212 98374 1

Printed in the Republic of Ireland
by HELY THOM LIMITED, Dublin.

Contents

Plates

Plates

VIII

The author and publisher wish to thank the following for their kind permission to use the plates in this book: *Professor Antonio Beltrán of Zarogoza University*—plate 3; *Archico Historico de Cerverea (Lerida)*—plate 7; *Biblioteca Nacional, Madrid*—plates 6, 9–13, 15, 17, 23, 26, 27, 29–31, 33–8, 43–61; *the Curator, Salisbury Cathedral*—plate 8; *Museo del Teatro, Madrid*—plates 14, 16; *Gyenes, Madrid*—plates 22, 62, 63, 68–70; *Victoria and Albert Museum, London*—plates 24, 25; *Harvard Theatre*—plates 39–42; Antonio—plates 64, 65.

Introduction

WHY IS it that so little has been written in the English language on the subject of Spanish dancing, with reference to its historical background? Could it be that we only like to watch and not to read about it? Are the movements so complex and the castanet rhythms so intricate that the limitation of words makes it impossible to describe them? Possibly, but this hardly explains why there is such a dearth of literature on Spanish dance history at a time when dance audiences everywhere are unusually well versed in that pertaining to other forms of dancing—thanks to the many treatises now in circulation. This book is in reality a modest attempt to remedy this deficiency.

Spanish dancing nowadays attracts larger audiences than in pre-war years and its popularity extends far beyond the boundaries of Spain. It is easy to guess why, where there are large colonies of people of Spanish descent as for example in America—Central, North and South. To see Spanish dances brings them nearer to the land of their forefathers, satisfying that infinite yearning for the mother country experienced by most Spaniards abroad. What is not so easy to account for is the impact Spanish dancing makes upon the audiences in Africa, Australia, Asia and India. That it exists is witnessed by the fact that Spanish companies touring these far-flung continents return home time and again, triumphantly success-ful, both from an artistic as well as a financial point of view.

As for Europe, most opera houses possess a resident ballet company where Spanish dance influence has made itself felt. These ballet groups nearly always include full-length ballets in their repertoires based on Spanish themes and also suites of Spanish dances. In very recent years, Antonio was engaged to produce Spanish ballets at the opera houses of Milan and Vienna to name but two, and only previous engagements prevented him from mounting the *Three-Cornered Hat* for the Ankara Ballet Company in Turkey.

There is nothing new in this. With the passage of time Spanish dance material has become closely woven into the fabric of classical ballet all over the world and, thus, Spain has made an impressive contribution to this international cause. As we shall see, ballet masters of the past discovered a fecund source of inspiration for their works in Spanish dancing. Although Spanish themes may not be quite so fashionable as a vehicle for full-length ballets as they were a hundred years ago, Spanish dancing in itself has become a strong enough force to hold its own in modern theatres—and fill them.

The curious paradox, however, is that despite this world-wide demand for Spanish ballet, Madrid today is the only European capital without an opera house or other large theatre especially devoted to the production of ballet. How is this possible in a country like Spain that, as far back as the eighteenth century, possessed a flourishing 'school' of academic classical dancing of its own, and whose people possess an inborn genius for dancing? What has happened to this inherited dance tradition? What prevents the appearance of a Spanish national ballet company in Madrid today?

Thereby hangs a long story. In an endeavour to find the answers to these and other equally tantalizing questions it will be necessary to touch upon the past. The present situation can only be attributed to the result of historical experience. History can only be written after delving into national records which, in turn, need to be carefully examined. Such documents have to be tracked down and are not always easy to come by. Many still lie hidden in private houses and public institutions to which ordinary readers may find some difficulty in gaining access. Quite a lot has inevitably been lost in the turmoils of war and national upheavals.

Now that public attention is focused on the building of a modern national theatre in Madrid destined to be devoted to opera, drama and ballet, it would appear that the time is ripe for such material as is available to be assembled.

Quite by chance, I was engaged to transform a Spanish folk-dancing group into a ballet company and so had the opportunity of working with Spanish dancers. Mentioning to Cyril Beaumont the dearth of literature on the history of Spanish dancing, he suggested that I was the person to write a concise history of Spanish dancing. This, however, turns out to be something of a 'publisher's risk' and so this book has been produced in a form suitable not only for dancers but also for general readers.

For almost eight years, whilst initiating the Dancing Spaniards into the mysteries of classical ballet technique, my contact with them was very personal and direct. Working with them day and night, I came to know them well, and as time went by my admiration for their inherited talent for dancing increased. Writing and research had to be fitted in between classes and rehearsals and proved to be a most enjoyable form of relaxation. After all, if one is not a writer in the professional sense, this is the sort of book that can be written for pleasure. It was never intended to be the definitive book on the history of Spanish dance for which the world is waiting. My professional commitments as ballet mistress precluded me from finding the time to disentangle the maze of dance material I found, with the thoroughness required for such a task. It is for others, better qualified than myself, to take up where I have left off and fill in the gaps. If this work proves to be no more than a point of departure for them, it will have served a most useful purpose.

What is Spanish Ballet?

BALLET AS now presented to Spanish audiences is a very different thing from that introduced by the Italians to eighteenth-century Spain. Ever since the Opera House closed in 1925, Madrid has been deprived of any sort of permanent ballet organization. As a result, numerous Spanish dance groups, large and small, regional, classical, or flamenco, came into existence, all styling themselves 'Ballet Español'. These have served to distort the original balletic form and the time seems to be ripe for a recall to Spanish Classical Ballet if, as is frequently reiterated, the new Spanish National Theatre which is intended to be a permanent organization, is really about to come into being.

For some time past, most Spaniards have agreed that the formation of a Spanish National Theatre is long overdue, but they talk about their opera and ballet as though it were a foregone conclusion! The fact that ballet as an art form took a long time to develop, and will take at least an equal amount to revive, appears to be overlooked. To build a magnificent modern theatre is not enough unless, at the same time, adequate preparations are made to train a company worthy to grace such a theatre.

What is now known as 'Russian Ballet' started by being French, then absorbed Italian influences, incorporated Isadora Duncan's concepts and also drew upon an apparently limitless repertoire of folk steps which were elaborated and slowly evolved into what we see today. This process of assimilation has been going on for centuries. In Russia, dancers had splendid training schools, a permanent theatre in which to dance, and, in the case of choreographers, to experiment in. Building up such a fabric entailed the expenditure of much money and a considerable amount of effort. It also called for a great deal of foresight on the part of many generations of artists of every kind, from many lands. A theatre is but the essential shell of a ballet, the kernel is the structure within, and this cannot germinate overnight.

Fortunately, Spain possesses a classical tradition of her own but she deviated from it at a time when the rest of Europe was busy developing theatrical dancing out of social dancing. In the eighteenth century, when the best dancing in Spain ceased to be performed at court by the leisured classes who had the time and money to cultivate it, professional dancing, as we shall see, was handed over to foreigners. This prevented any direct transition from social to Spanish stage dancing. Theatrical dancing was influenced by the Italians and social dancing by the French, while Spanish dancing was left to the lower orders and accordingly came to be despised by the Spanish upper classes. The notable exception was the bolero, which the Italians had taken and cleverly moulded into a balletic shape. They accomplished this so successfully that it became the main feature of solo dancing when the Spanish theatre was established. The brilliant execution of these elaborate steps by Spanish dancers attracted foreigners from other lands, who copied them.

A codified system of teaching dancing then existed in Spain, out of which grew a tradition which powerfully influenced nineteenth-century European choreography. In the present century, however, Spanish dancers show signs of turning their backs upon this heritage. If the new theatre were to be opened tomorrow, the only types of Spanish dancing ready to be presented on the stage are flamenco and regional, neither of which is an essentially theatrical form of dancing.

Historical writings still in existence, which are mentioned later, prove that a whole store of information on dance form was available in the seventeenth and eighteenth centuries. Suites of dances have been left, recorded for future choreographers to use, and the Spanish dancing masters clearly explained their mode of teaching. There was no doubt about how to strengthen the feet in those days: instep control was the answer. Nor could there by any question about the

2

form of a dance, for the diagrams made the pattern of the master's choreography obvious at once. This was how technique was built up in Spain—as indeed it was everywhere else at the same period, renslting in the sort of classical ballet instruction given in ballet schools nowadays all over the world. This classical ballet technique is still adapted to present-day requirements, with the most interesting results, in all the large national training schools attached to state-subsidized theatres.

In the light of modern knowledge, there is no reason why a twentieth-century Spanish Bolero School should not outshine anything which has gone before. Yet, the sad fact is, that inside Spain, if a student wished to study Spanish classical dancing with the same degree of thoroughness as classical ballet is studied elsewhere in Europe, it would be very hard indeed to find a school specializing in this type of instruction. Nowadays, a pupil can pick up a bolero along with a jota, a fandango and the sevillanas at any *academía* but that is as far as it goes.

The great dancers directing their own companies do their best to conserve what remains of the old 'Spanish School' for they realize its value, but it plays a minor part in their repertoire since international audiences do not share their interest. With so much dance material within Spain it would be easy to build up a good repertoire choreographically, but the backbone of any good company is a first-class *corps de ballet*, technically equipped to carry out the ideas of the choreographers and this seems to be what is lacking.

At present, the Spaniards are working in reverse, or so it seems to anyone accustomed to working in an orthodox ballet company. They are trying to impose classical technique upon adult folk dancers who, in any other country, would be considered too mature to start serious balletic training. It is interesting to observe that, when these trials are made, the dancers themselves perceive that a strong classical foundation must be laid before attempting to incorporate their own folk idiom into theatrical dancing. The present state of dancing in Spain indicates a grave doubt as to whether the dancing Spaniards of today would have the stamina to sustain a full-length ballet as had their forebears in the past. No doubt, once the theatre is established in Madrid, the lessons of the past will be

3

learnt and inspiration sought in the works left by the old Spanish masters, so that ultimately a new tradition will emerge, built on the foundation already laid. If only as a museum piece, a five-act Spanish ballet would be a revelation to the modern world.

It might be as well to digress for a moment to consider what is meant in Spain today by 'ballet español', for it may help us to understand how the present situation has come about. Before the Teatro Real closed down in Madrid, regular seasons of opera and ballet were given there and ballet had the same significance for Spaniards up to the early 1920s as it has now for most people in Western Europe. That this is no longer the case in Spain, is probably due to the fact that going to the 'Real' was not only an artistic experience, but also a social event, enjoyed by the royal and every other family. The passing of one has meant the disappearance of the other.

Up to the time of the Spanish Civil War, Spanish dancing was chiefly confined to cabarets, café chantants, or vaudeville; folk-dancing flourished in the countryside. After the Civil War was over, a very determined effort was made to put Spanish dancing of all kinds into the theatre and this became particularly noticeable after the Second World War. Great efforts have been made both in America and Europe and they have been successful up to a point, although nothing in the nature of a three-act ballet has yet emerged. It follows from this, that when a Spaniard refers to a 'ballet', he does not mean what others understand by ballet, for his mind conjures up a group of people doing Spanish dancing anywhere. The curious thing is that although ballet as an art form has disappeared from the Spanish scene, the word has not. Spaniards still use this foreign term, in a different sense, and they pronounce it differently, sounding the final 't'.

In modern Spanish a *danza* or a *baile* is a dance and the verb *danzar* and *bailar* express the act of dancing. Yet, this was not always so, for in earlier days a clear distinction was made between the two. As far back as 1635, Gonzalez de Sales explained that a *danza* consisted of more measured movements than a *baile*, only the feet were used and the arms were kept quite still. Skill was required to perform a *danza* well, and this necessitated the service of a specialized teacher. Since the study of *danzas* was reserved for the higher orders, society accepted them, indeed to excel in them was considered the height of social distinction.

By contrast, a *baile* was conspicuous by the freedom of movement displayed; particularly movements of the head, body and arms. It was usually of a collective nature, performed by a number of people and generally referred to a folk-dance. At the same period, a *baile* was also the term applied to a literary form, consisting of little sketches and plays dealing with dancing as a theme. Dancing schools and dancing masters became favourite topics during the seventeenth century and Quiñoñes de Benevente was but one author who wrote prolifically and excelled in this type of work.

With the passage of time, a strange thing has happened, for the meaning of the words has been reversed; a *baile* is now a *danza* and vice versa and this should not be forgotten when trying to fit Spanish ballet into the modern background. Today, Spaniards speak about *baile clásico* or *danzas de España*—the latter being the folk dances o Spain. There is an officially sponsored company, for example, called 'Coros y Danzas de España' doing magnificent work in bringing authentic regional dances to the notice of foreign audiences (pl. 62). *Baile clásico* is no other than Spanish classical dancing of the highly developed bolero school.

With this fundamental change of conception concerning the native dances, it is hardly surprising to find that the balletic content of 'Ballet Español' has diminished to such an extent that it no longer bears any resemblance to ballet as generally understood by other European audiences. Yet, while retaining the foreign term 'ballet', the Spaniards have dropped the foreign title of 'ballerina', preferring to use the Spanish *bailarina* or *bailadora* when referring to a dancer, but they differentiate between these, too. A *bailadora* refers to a gypsy dancer whether a born gypsy or not; one who dances in the streets or 'dives' for gain. A *bailarina* on the other hand, is one who studies the art of dancing, to perform either in an amateur or professional capacity in the theatre or ballroom. The underlying nuance appears to be that the first consists of instinctive dancing while the other is an acquired knowledge of the art. This modern distinction is closely related to the seventeenth-century conception of *danzar* and *bailar* with all the social implications involved. The meaning may seem complicated to foreigners but it is quite clear to a Spaniard who is accustomed to use these terms in everyday conversation. Real confusion arises only when the non-Spanish term 'ballet' is employed, for the majority of Spanish people understand it to mean group dancing as opposed to solo dancing—Spanish dancing of course.

At this point, it might be as well to consider what 'ballet' means outside Spain, for some may think that nowadays it is a somewhat ambiguous term everywhere! True, it may refer to various aspects of choreographic art, ranging from pornographic gymnastics to the most abstract psychological conception of movement. It may also represent nothing more than a form of technique couched in French terms. 'Classical ballet technique' refers to a type of technique that came into being in the seventeenth century. Influenced by the French and Italians in their midst at that time, Spanish technique developed along similar lines until the late eighteenth century when it began to show marked national characteristics, spreading in the nineteenth century to countries outside Spain, where it was adopted and thereby influenced European theatrical choreography.

There is a tendency to confuse 'ballet—divertissement' with ballet. A work which consists of joining dances together into a suite of dances is often called a ballet, although there is no story attached to it. the time value may be that of a single act in a complete ballet, but this is in fact a 'divertissement' and nearly all programmes of Spanish ballet today are made up entirely of divertissements; they form the nucleus of every repertory in the Spanish 'cuadros' abroad and are very popular in Spain.

Quite a number of ballet lovers regard ballet as nothing more than a name given to an organization that stages ballets, and to them 'going to the ballet' means no more than patronizing their own favourite company—rather like football fans who go to cheer their home team. By and large, a ballet company of this kind consists of a highly organized body of trained dancers, musicians, scenic artists, designers, producers, choreographers, stage technicians and all the paraphernalia of administration. A great deal of money is required to maintain it which is far beyond the means of private individuals today. This type of company usually receives a grant from the state or from a foundation. It may be a royal, national or democratic institution with headquarters in the capital city. Attached to the company is an equally highly-organized training school, destined to give an adequate artistic and general education to the young aspirants who hope to become the dance artists of the future. At the moment of writing, nothing of this kind exists in Spain.

As for the ballet itself, it may consist of two or three acts, even four may sometimes be seen. When, in the past, the possibilities of producing ballet in Spain were explored, grandiose ballets modelled on Noverre lines resulted and the Spaniards distinguished themselves by producing five-act ballets. Compared with present-day standards, this was no mean feat, for in those days, each act contained more than one scene. If any eighteenth-century Spanish balletomane felt the urge to applaud the legendary hero of chivalry, Don Quixote, in balletic form, he could do so, in old Madrid. Compare the position with the present, when if, by some remote chance, a modern Spaniard felt inclined to indulge this whim, he would have to go to Russia, China or England to satisfy it! Since nothing remains of these classics in Spain, what has replaced them?

In recent years the most interesting productions from a balletic point of view have been undoubtedly the works mounted by Spanish companies directed by Spanish dancers of international repute such as Pilar Lopez, Mariemma, El Greco, Antonio and Lusillio, who dance the leading roles in them. They are the only people in a position to make choreographic experiments but, since there is insufficient work to keep them busy inside Spain all the year round, they can scarcely be considered part of the Spanish dancing scene. Their survival depends upon long lucrative tours abroad and, accordingly, their repertoires are designed for foreign taste rather than Spanish. Madrid and Barcelona may have the chance of seeing them before they set off on their travels for a brief season—perhaps once every two years, but no more. The productions are prepared with great care; well-known artists are commissioned to design scenery and costumes and intricate lighting plots are evolved to implement often elaborate choreographic creations. There is an international flavour about these troupes because not all the members are Spaniards. In recent years, much energy has been expended trying to convert folk-dancing groups into ballet companies in the international sense and they are becoming 'Ballet Español' at its biggest and most experimental best; rarely seen in Spain and not always appreciated. The only really permanent dance spectacles there are those given by the small troupes of 'Ballet Español' which are featured in Spanish operettas, vaudeville and music halls.

These ambitious companies run on a big scale and, mounted by world famous Spanish dancers, do not content themselves with Spanish dancing alone; they show a keen desire to produce Spanish ballet in as complete a theatrical form as possible and, bearing in mind the limited means at their disposal, they succeed very well. Musically, they follow the formula laid down in the 1930s by La Argentina. Credit must be accorded to that great artist for having revealed the possibilities of interpreting Spanish classical music through the medium of theatrical dancing. This was revolutionary at the time, particularly when she took the works of Albeniz, Granados, de Falla, Turina, Halffter and translated them into terms of Spanish dancing which she staged magnificently, sparing no expense on costumes and scenery, and so produced twentieth-century Spanish ballet. The artistic calendar of the Paris Opera House or the Opéra Comique was never complete without a season of Spanish ballet given by Argentina. Versatile, she was equally at home on large opera house stages or in the concert hall, where she gave dance recitals with only a concert pianist and her castanets to accompany her. As Segovia transformed the guitar into a concert instrument, so did Argentina transform the castanets. Fired by her virtuosity, young dance students took up the castanets, not with any idea of becoming Spanish dancers, but from the sheer joy of listening to her records and trying to emulate her virtuosity. It all sounded so simple, easy and flowing. As for her danced creations, they combined mimed movement with stylized steps and, for the most part, were confined to solos and suites of dances. Argentina gave the message of Spanish dancing to the world in a highly individualized personal manner. Her productions were in impeccable taste in every detail and she elevated Spanish dancing to a theatrical art of the highest quality, thereby proving that Spanish dancing could be transplanted into the modern theatre and successfully developed into Spanish ballet.

Born of Spanish parents in Buenos Aires, La Argentina was destined to reveal to the world through Spanish masterpieces the great power of dancing. Argentina's success in the present century recalls the services rendered to the cause of Spanish dancing in the past by Fanny Elslser, curiously enough, again like Argentina, also at the Paris Opera House. The constant resurgence of Spanish theatrical dancing frequently appears to take place abroad, and when this happens it becomes so fashionable that it borders on mania. The main hindrance to progress inside Spain always seems to have been caused by the deep-rooted social prejudice the Spaniards have against theatrical dancing generally. Since the Second World War, there has been an increasing tendency in those European countries where large government subsidies finance national schools of ballet, to consider ballet theatres important to the artistic culture of the nations, placed on a similar level as art galleries, libraries and museums. In England, the habit of going to the ballet is being inculcated in the young by giving them the opportunity of seeing special school performances within school hours. These are in the nature of lessons in ballet appreciation. The children are told the story of the ballet, they learn that as in opera and drama a ballet is composed of acts, usually two or three, and finally, the object is to tell a story, with movement as a mode of expression, just as in drama, words, and in opera, song, are used as a vehicle. They realize that the mission of dancers is to express emotion and interpret musical composition through mime, gesture and movement, and this is the way in which the audiences of tomorrow are formed. This cannot happen in the Peninsula until some sort of officially-sponsored ballet comes into existence. Argentina prepared the ground artistically, showing how Spanish dancing lends itself to balletic interpretation; it remains for the Spaniards to do the rest.

Her major works were the great revelation of the 1930s. *El Amor Brujo* was one—this work had been originally composed for the superb Spanish artist, Pastora Imperio. In 1935, La Argentina, supported by her own company, took Paris by storm with her interpretation. Later, her triumphant world tours enabled audiences to hear Spanish music hitherto rarely, if ever, heard outside Spain and certainly not in the theatre. Halffter's *Sonatina* and de Falla's *La Vida Breve* and *El Amor Brujo* were but a few of these early pioneering efforts.

It is this initial spade work which has helped Spanish dancers in modern times to develop their dancing further along theatrical lines. Using original choreography, they have made a synthesis of folk and classical dancing in the Spanish manner and evolved it to a still higher degree of perfection. The production side has improved enormously, since great strides in the technique of theatre lighting have been made everywhere during the past thirty years. After Argentina's death however, the dances of Spain seemed to return to the cafés, cabarets and night clubs (pl. 63).

While Spain was in the grip of the Civil War, her dancing survived by being conserved beyond the frontiers of the Peninsula. As Spanish refugees poured out of Spain, they were obliged to find a means of earning a living and many solved the problem by dancing in public—a thing they would not have dreamed of doing before the war. In the principal European cities, the bars, cabarets, music halls and concert halls—where there were any—were soon peopled by Spanish dance groups. They superseded the waves of Russian dancers who had previously built a reputation, in similar haunts and for the same reason. Spanish cabaret and dance recitals became the vogue but the style of Spanish dancing then was not what we see today, for fashions in dancing also change. The favourite type of dancing most commonly seen in those days was either of the Spanish classical or regional variety; flamenco was a rarity. Indeed it was only after the Second World War, that flamenco dancing became popular and flamenco-mania rampant. The enormous popularity of Spanish gypsy dancing may well be the reason why Spanish classical dancing has receded into the background. One of the most noticeable things about the repertories of Spanish dance groups today is the small percentage of classical dancing contained in them and this is true, both in and outside Spain. When a Spanish company produces work of a classical nature nowadays, the tendency is to turn towards unfamiliar classical ballet technique for inspiration, instead of Spanish classical dancing of the Bolero School which the Spaniards know so well.

Regional dancing has lost none of its attraction and it gains in favour year by year in Spanish dance groups, both large and small. Suites of dances from the various regions are always sure of certain success. The wholesale invasion of the theatre by regional dancing is a post-war innovation, by no means peculiar to Spain. London, Paris and the other capital cities of the world possessing a large ballet-going public are rarely without some nationally-sponsored folk-dance company and it may be supposed that in this matter Spain is just following the general trend. Nevertheless, it is difficult to understand why, in the domain of Spanish dancing, flamenco and regional dancing—neither of which is theatrical in origin—should be so popular in the theatre, whereas Spanish classical dancing, which was primarily developed as a theatrical form in the eighteenth century, should be neglected. Dance recitals of this kind have become almost obsolete in recent years, but like some rare museum object, one is suddenly produced, usually by a member of that unique Spanish classical dancing family, Pericet.

A link with the past is that most Spanish dance groups of international fame are usually directed by Spanish women; Pilar Lopez, Mariemma, the late Carmen Amaya, Rosario spring to mind at once, but only one group is run by a Spanish man and that is the company headed by Antonio. All the other male directors are either North or Latin Americans and they add to their conception of Spanish dancing, foreign standards of production, interesting to foreign audiences but not always to the taste of the Spanish, who tend to criticise their innovations harshly.

All the great Spanish directors who have succeeded in forming their own companies tour abroad, and during their travels have the chance of seeing modern and classical ballets in the international sense. This has given them some insight into the way in which to run a ballet company and they try to apply this knowledge to the running of their own companies. Elements from foreign choreography are used but with discretion, for they have to be in keeping with contemporary Spanish taste for there are still many Spaniards who like their Spanish dancing unadulterated. In spite of many obstacles, these pioneers are doing wonderful work in placing such Spanish ballet as there is—as opposed to Spanish dancing—on the map, and that is about all that can be done for the moment.

The chief obstacle to sustained progress is lack of adequate funds to keep a company running all the year round. If a Spanish ballet company suffers a loss, it is at once dissolved and the members seek work elsewhere and are lost forever to the original company which had given them enough training to be useful to it. All the privately-run dance groups lack stability, because there are no impressarios forthcoming of the Diaghleff, de Cuevas category, willing to devote their private fortunes to financing Spanish ballet. This means that Spanish companies are always on the point of forming, disbanding or reforming; new members have to be brought in to replace those who have gone and with a constantly changing *corps de ballet* which has to be trained as they work, any possibility of producing any sort of ensemble or improving the standard of the dancing is very slight.

As a rule, a company will start very well with all the dancers wildly enthusiastic, as only Spaniards know how to be. Every member is an eager crusader in the great cause of Spanish dance. They all put their hearts into what they are doing; patriotism is never very far from their dancing—as much a reality today as ever it was in the past. Indeed this appears to be the main driving force as all the warmth, vitality and love of country inherent in that very inflammable entity '*el alma español*' is there plain for all to see. As rehearsals proceed, the dancers appear to weary, the crusading spirit to wilt and things begin to go very wrong. It would be foolish to pretend that restlessness only exists in Spanish companies for this is common to most ballet groups; outside Spain, it is never allowed to interfere with the discipline of the company. Not so in the case of the Spanish dancers, who show their discontent, often by grumbling like small children, making exaggerated demands for more money; at times, absenteeism replaces the former keenness and idealism. Everything suddenly seems to be overshadowed by a feeling of mistrust for all direction. The dancers, who are not used to working so hard for any length of time, feel that unreasonable demands are made upon them, which they resent. This poses the question: how can this lack of 'conditioning' to theatrical needs be remedied? The obvious answer is of course, training—but where is this to be found?

Within my experience, Spanish dancers differ from those in the theatres of other countries by the fact that in most cases they have had no theatrical training whatsoever, and in many cases they had never set foot on a stage in their lives. It was not surprising therefore that they found it hard to understand why they had to rehearse once they had learnt the dance sequence, and the daily routine of class and rehearsal was far beyond their comprehension! They indignantly maintained that they knew how to dance and had no need to 'learn' and what was more, with their independent spirit, they were not prepared to follow anyone, or keep in line with their colleagues, either! To ask them to do so, they considered a gross interference with their personal liberty!

The fact is, Spanish dancers are not slavish copyists which, artistically, is a valuable quality in itself provided it is coupled with theatrical knowledge. They have an unusual capacity for absorbing movements not their own and transmuting them into something quite different. When this is properly directed it will be of great advantage, but meanwhile it is only a hindrance. Indeed, this is the major problem confronting anyone trying to form a company and striving for some sort of unity or uniformity of movement. It will never be solved until every single member of the company realizes that he has to be as good in his own department as is the first dancer in his or hers. This state of mind has yet to be cultivated.

With the world-wide demand for Spanish dancing, the young Spaniards now have the opportunity to travel and learn, as their leaders have learned, how dance artists in other countries are formed. They can see for themselves how slowly and seriously dance students work in the classrooms. Slowly they are beginning to perceive that instinct for dancing is not enough in the theatre. They cannot put into practice this new discovery, however, until they too will in the future have the chance to work regularly in the theatre, instead of just dabbling in it for a few months every year.

They have already proved that they have dance instinct in abundance, when they confine themselves to their own dances, but they become too painfully aware of their limitations when they branch out into other forms of dancing. In small groups, lack of stage-craft and ensemble or technical weaknesses are not very noticeable but when the small group is expanded into a big company, these defects become visible at once.

There are so few large companies in Spain, that they have never had to preoccupy themselves with these things. Slowly now, the Spanish dancers are becoming aware of them and the feeling is growing that there ought to be some training centres in Spain where those who aspire to become dancers may receive proper instruction, an adequate general education, a knowledge of stage-craft, a grounding in ballet technique, combined with a complete study of Spanish dancing in all its aspects. Many of the dancers already dream of the day when they will know as much about classical ballet as they do about their own dancing. The girls in particular are especially attracted to it. Meanwhile, most Spanish dancers just have to be content with the modest groups of 'ballet español' which perform in Spain all the year round and form the only training ground they know.

From a serious, professional point of view, the training obtainable in Spain at present seems to be somewhat haphazard. Really hard work in the classroom is unheard of, silence is emphatically not golden—and chatter disturbs anybody accustomed to working in the claustral silence of a ballet classroom. Choreology is at present unknown. This situation is unimportant as long as there is no national ballet organiaztion demanding an annual intake of new talent, to realize the projects of the following season. The fact that there is no rallying ground, in the form of a subsidized headquarters, is quite enough to explain the average Spanish dancer's attitude.

As individuals, Spanish dancers are hot-tempered, charming, quick-witted, fiercely jealous of their colleagues and, as a result, frequently on the defensive. Never having been through 'school' they have no cause to suppress their emotions and so, when they dance, they feel their way emotionally, rather than by reasoning. They know how to love, how to hate, how to feel deeply; they explain solemnly and in all sincerity that their dancing comes from the soul—*el alma español*. The Spanish dancer convinces himself that thinking about dancing is going to interfere with the free play of his imagination and claims that he cannot work like other people, so it is wasting his time to work in a studio. He may well be right and, given this mental approach, this is certainly true at present.

Despite these pronouncements, it should not be thought that there are no studios in Spain. There are many in all the big cities and there is a wide variety from which to choose. The shrines of flamenco in Madrid are often of the 'hole in the wall' variety, with rickety floors, quite airless and accordingly rather pungent; freezing in the winter, stifling in the summer. They are much sought after by the foreigners because they measure up to their conception of Spanish 'local colour' which they feel aids them in mastering this elusive style of Spanish dancing. The students, like the swallows, return regularly every year and some remain for months on end. Spanish dancers also attend these classes, many of them relatives of the teacher, for the Spanish dancing 'clan' is vast. Others go only for brief periods, enough time in which to learn a dance or two, to get a job in a night club.

There is also a vogue for practising flamenco as a hobby among the aristocracy and, as in the seventeenth century, they usually study in the privacy of their own homes, where the teacher visits them, bringing a guitarrist to accompany or, occasionally, performing this office himself.

The nearest approach to a professional training centre is to be found in a block of ancient studios in the poetically named Street of God's Love (Amor de Dios) situated in old Madrid. The odd thing about the classes here is that none of the people who attend them has been artistically formed since childhood by the teacher. Despairingly, the instructors complain that it is not worth their while exhausting themselves in making corrections, since nobody ever studies with them for long. These studios are otherwise similar to those at the Dance Centre in Floral Street, Covent Garden, London, or the Salle Wacker in Paris, for they are hired out by the hour to singers, dancers and musicians. Here it is that the agents seek members for their cabaret acts, extras for the many foreign films now being made in Spain, and for the 'Cuadros' of 'Ballet Español'.

Open classes are held there daily at a set hour, by the same teacher. The atmosphere is delightfully convivial and informal; as in the eighteenth-century bolero studies, there is plenty of smoke— only not coming from cigars but from the cigarettes smoked by the many spectators who crowd the room to watch the class. Naturally, these people could not be expected to keep silent very long and in addition to talking among themselves, they chat to the waiters who come in from a nearby café bearing trays of beer, wine, prawns and other such titbits to nibble with the drinks. Between sips and nibbles, fond parents may be heard to throw out a word of encouragement or criticism to their offspring at the *barre*, or even proffer a word of advice to the teacher! Their voices have to be raised to be heard above the din of the piano accompaniment! But teacher and pupils take it all in their stride, as they plod through a ballet barre, with some limbering added, and go into the centre, to perform a strange medley of modern, classical, acrobatic and Spanish steps. Pirouettes are practised with the dancers playing their castanets. The lesson concludes with a figure from one of the traditional Spanish dances.

Many foreign dancers attend these classes, often the girls from the troupes appearing in revues and night clubs. The Spanish dancers are nearly always those from the 'Ballet Español' groups who go in the hope of picking up another job while at the same time keeping in trim. These classes are in reality organized practices. Little or no correction is given and the dancers, like the spectators, chat among themselves as they work and appear thoroughly to enjoy themselves.

There is a third type of studio, although not concerned with the training of professional dancers, which is nevertheless important when considering Spanish ballet as a whole. This kind of academy is very clean, well ventilated, situated in the modern part of Madrid, often in the elegant modern blocks of flats in the smart suburbs. These studios cater for the wealthy amateurs and their children who will be the audiences of the future. The instruction is quite unpretentious, because the pupils look down upon the theatre to such an extent that the mere idea of entering it as a profession fills them only with amusement or horror. They dance purely for pleasure, learning a little Spanish dancing, and some modern and classical ballet. The instruction given in these studios is often very sound as far as it goes, for the teacher has probably studied abroad. Often the daughter of middle-class parents, the instructress, not being permitted to follow up her foreign training by dancing in the theatre, as the next best thing, opens her own studio. It is quite respectable to teach, though not to dance in public, in Madrid.

The social stigma that is still attached to dancing on the stage in Spain, surprises anybody coming from countries where such dancing is considered an accepted profession. The flat refusal of Spanish parents to allow their daughters to take up professional dancing may be traced to the current practice of religious dancing, still to be seen in religious processions and inside churches. The 'Seises' still perform their famous figure dance before the High Altar in Seville Cathedral, said to be in memory of David dancing before the Ark. According to Garcia Matos,[1] dancing was used in the Corpus processions as a direct result of a pronouncement by Pope Urbano IV. The custom spread and has continued to take place in all Spanish regions in the present day. 'Gigantones' are as much a part of religious processions as they were in the past. Miniature pantomimes take place, when children will gleefully enter the giant's mouth to be gobbled up, slither though his interior to emerge from the other end with delighted gurgles. In this context, this sort of performance is taken quite seriously in Spain and so are performances of jotas, fandangos and seguidillas on the threshold of the church—danced in a spirit of devout homage. But when similar dances are put on to public platforms, in theatres and cabarets, they come in for criticism on moral grounds. Attention is drawn to the erotic, sensuous and voluptuous qualities then considered to be inherent in the dances. Spanish moralists are even now preoccupied with the question of morality in dancing and write on the subject. As yet, no satisfactory answer has been found

[1]M. Garcia Matos: *Veijas canciones y melodías en la musica instrumental popular de las danzas procesionales practicadas aûn en España.* (Consejo superior de investigaciones cientificas—Barcelona 1958–61).

to this traditionally Spanish problem which ultimately will have to be solved by the Spaniards themselves, in as Spanish a manner as possible, if ever the magnificent dancing heritage bequeathed to the Spaniards is to be successfully harnessed, without prejudice, to the fundamental needs of the new national ballet.

While dancing in modern Spain continues to be considered the Cinderella of the arts, it will go on stagnating in the 'cuadros' of the night clubs, music halls and operettas. The repertoire varies but little from that of the last century in similar haunts, except that the 'cuadro bolero' has become almost obsolete, having been replaced by the 'cuadro flamenco'. Before the Civil War, a 'cuadro bolero' would function side by side with a 'cuadro flamenco'. The artists in one were quite separate from the other, and both cuadros were equally popular. In those days, the women dancers spent the day looking after the children, doing their washing and housework and then went off to the café at night to earn extra money. In 1961, a night club in Madrid revived the custom, by featuring two 'cuadros'. It was a successful experiment and pleased all who visited the place. The 'cuadro bolero', attired in eighteenth-century 'majo' costumes, were accompanied by musicians similarly attired in rich satins of delicate apple green and pale rose pink. They performed on a tiny platform and, after the fire and frenzy of the flamenco group which preceded them, they appeared so elegantly refined by contrast, that they might have stepped straight out of the courtly times of Carlos III.

The 'cuadros' or 'Ballet Español' groups are not preceded by clever public relations or elaborate publicity on a big scale. A simple poster or announcement in the daily press makes it known where they are to be found. It may read something like this: 'Parma Violet, and her famous Ballet Español, appears nightly at . . .' and that may mean anything from a group of two to twenty-two. Unpretentious as a rule, without décor, but with a blinding light from one or two projectors and, of course, no orchestra. To compensate for these deficiencies, there is plenty of 'atmosphere' which consists of making as much noise as possible. Finger-snapping, heel-stamping, foot-tapping, crackling castanets with the monotonous wailing of the 'cantaor'. This helps to satisfy the kind of public that has come to expect the maximum amount of noise from any company calling itself Spanish. The guitarrists mitigate the racket by their quota of soothing strumming and are remarkable for their odd names which, when translated, mean 'Overcoat', 'Jacket', or even 'Trousers', following the gypsy custom of calling their singers and musicians after wearing apparel. The 'ballet' is expected to dance on a handkerchief of a floor, or a tiny platform, but no matter how modest the group, the dancers are invariably well groomed and beautifully tailored. The programme consists of classical, regional and flamenco dancing. Leaps, turns and acrobatic feats are sometimes added as a novelty and whatever the dance, it is usually exaggerated—the flamenco excessively fiery, the classical trimmed with stunts. It is interesting to observe how the dancers in these small groups follow the example of the choreographers in larger companies, by mixing Spanish dancing with such widely divergent types of movement as jazz, ye-ye, or ballet. The young Spanish dancers appear to be fascinated by any sort of novelty and are always seeking new ways of presenting their dances. It would be an exaggeration to claim that pure Spanish dancing does not exist in these haunts for it does, but is mainly found in those in the smaller Spanish towns and in certain exclusively Spanish cabarets, unknown to the visitor. Most of the entertainment provided in the capital is intended for tourists and this description of 'Ballet Español' refers to the ever popular spectacles offered in Madrid, Barcelona and similar big cities as one of the highlights of night life.

One type of 'Ballet Español' fares somewhat better than the modest little duos, trios and quartets working in the 'cuadros' and those are the ballets included in the Spanish music-hall productions. The dancers are better off because the show runs all the year round and they are working under theatrical conditions with an adequate stage, where they have room to move, stage lighting and an orchestra. The Spanish dancing in this type of production is usually of the regional variety. The people responsible for the dance arrangements do not experiment, but use well-known jotas, fandangos or zapateados. The dancers are dressed in colourful costumes—of authentic design, as a rule. These shows correspond to the sort of musical comedies one sees in most capital cities. They provide the only permanent employment there is for dancers, of a theatrical nature, in Spain, as, once the season is over in Madrid, the company takes to the road and tours the smaller towns for the rest of the year, then returns once more to the capital with another production the following season. The Variety Theatre, too, provides some work for dancers, but it is mostly troupe work and Spanish dancers do not show up to the best advantage when herded together. The preference for bijou 'Ballet Español' really stems from the fact that in Madrid, at any rate, there is a dearth of big theatres.

In this respect, Barcelona fares better. The Catalans possess an ideal theatre for ballet production in the privately-owned Liceo. The seasons of opera and ballet there maintain the continuity for the old custom of 'going to the opera'. The city is close to the border and is easily accessible to foreign companies and therefore the inhabitants have a better chance of enjoying international opera and ballet than do the Madrileños. There is an officially-sponsored season held every year known as the *Festivales de Arte Teatrale*. Leading artists from various parts of the world usually make at least one appearance, in a repertoire of classical and modern works.

There is also a band of local artists attached to the Liceo but since the theatre is not open all the year round, they only appear intermittently. The fact that they have the chance to appear in the theatre regularly is a step in the right direction, for as yet no other group of the kind exists anywhere else in Spain. The immense stage at the Liceo is a glorious relic of an operatic past and the proscenium is said to be larger than that at the Scala, Milan. The front of the house is provided with tiers of cosy boxes, upholstered in warm red plush adorned with bobbles and the interior is handsomely decorated with paintings. Any artist who has appeared at the Liceo cherishes the warmest affection for this theatre with its faintly musty whiff of a romantic past. It is easy to recall memories of royal command performances, brilliant seasons of Russian ballet and, more recently, those of the incomparable Argentina. That great artist was held in such esteem by the Spaniards, that a special room is devoted to a collection of her belongings in the Theatre Museum, close by the Liceo. In days gone by, there was a fine airy room on the top floor where the ballet companies used to rehearse. The warm Spanish sun streamed through the windows to welcome the dancers and stimulate them in their morning exertions. That was in Pavlova's day. In Antonio's, which is the present, the dancers are relegated to the cavernous depths of the basement, possessing an aroma vaguely reminiscent of Etruscan tombs. It is in this windowless, airless, odoriferous room that Spanish dancers are expected to practise, rehearse and find inspiration. This presents a perfect symbol of the depths to which the art of the dance has sunk.

The daughter of a wealthy industrialist could dance at the Liceo and, although this is not yet usual, it could happen without the girl being regarded as some sort of monster with five heads, because she is a ballet dancer—as is the case in some parts of Spain. In days gone by, professional dancers were considered to be promiscuous in many places and were socially condemned, but during the past fifty years, this prejudice has abated in the rest of Europe although not quite in the Iberian Peninsula.

The habit of despising those who dance in the theatre has become ingrained in the Spaniards so that at present, no matter how much talent a well-born young girl might possess, her chances of developing it in the world of ballet are very remote indeed. Male dancers fare still worse because as elsewhere, unfortunately, they are socially suspect. No Spanish gentleman could become a dancer without losing caste, and it is most unlikely that the idea would even enter the average Spanish male's head.

Speaking generally, careers for girls are not yet fashionable although there are unmistakable signs that Spanish girls are now allowed more freedom than before and begin to feel the urge to be independent. Spanish girls who take jobs, do so as a rule, however, from financial necessity, rarely for fun as do the girls in other lands. As for the Spanish dancers, they appear to associate work with one thing only—poverty. They have told me that they dance primarily in order to live. Antonio, the most famous of all Spanish dancers today, is an example, for he has kept his family ever since he was eight years old. Having danced all his life, he can with truth write: 'To dance is to live and to live is to dance'.

Probably all the great Spanish dancers have perfected their art in this way. Dancing since childhood has disciplined them, but the same cannot be said about the majority of the members of Spanish ballet companies. These people have usually drifted into the theatre from other jobs, expecting to have an easier life there and earn more money. Many, after a hard childhood doing all manner of work, graduate into being waiters, porters, nurses or typists, all poorly-paid occupations in Spain until quite recently. The theatre to them presents the possibility of meeting someone rich, either to marry or simply to keep them and their families. Once these boys and girls are married and have children of their own, they rarely permit them to dance—not from any moral scruples, as is the case with the affluent Spanish families, but for purely practical reasons! They openly declare that having only danced in order to eat and having found it very hard work, they would never want their children to 'suffer' in this way! The more financially successful go a step further in discouraging their children from dancing, because now that they have the means they want them to be 'educated'; in their own words, to become 'Señoritas'—ladies—which means that they must go to school and study.

Spanish dancers seem to think that a 'lady' and a 'dancer' are two separate identities, one quite incompatible with the other, because one is educated and the other is not. They surprised me by their rooted conviction that if dancers were educated, their dancing would lose some of its *sal* or fire. An easy pronouncement to make and one that has been accepted for generations, but how can anyone judge in this day and age, until the experiment has been made? All these preconceived notions concerning dancers and dancing are bound up with traditional misgivings of a moral nature, simply because ballet in Spain is not yet considered to be either an educative force or a vocational career. Until this attitude changes, it is unlikely that the matter can progress very far. Many Spaniards assure one that things are changing, but if change there be, it is so slight as to be imperceptible to the outside observer.

Some efforts have been made in recent years to break down these age-old barriers and the lead has been taken by the leading Spanish dance artists themselves. Those with sufficient means have founded their own groups, always hoping that their company might be favoured with a grant and become a permanent one; essentially Spanish in style and temperament but based on a classical foundation—for their experience of the theatre had taught them that this discipline was the most complete one as yet, and therefore indispensable. Their groups were a notable feature of the international festivals of art during the summer months. They were a means by which the young dancers became accustomed to adapt themselves to unfamiliar stage surroundings, and they gave them an opportunity to gain experience touring. They were also useful in helping to consolidate their repertory of classical, regional and contemporary works during a season of the year when it is notoriously difficult everywhere for ballet companies to obtain engagements. As the years have gone by, it has become obvious that the leaders, far from achieving their objective of founding something permanent, are severely handicapped by insufficient numbers of classically trained dancers staying with them long enough to realize their ever-increasingly ambitious choreographic creations, and so each year their experimental work is brought to an abrupt standstill.

Enough has been said to indicate the state of 'Ballet Español' today and to show the manifold difficulties at present impeding any further growth. The continual lack of understanding with which the vast majority of Spaniards approach theatrical dancing represents the major obstacle to making any lasting improvement in the standard of Spanish ballet today. The future of 'Ballet Español' appears to be at the crossroads and any further developments will be in the hands of the dancing Spaniards of tomorrow. How much progress they will make depends largely on how long they have to wait for their permanent theatre in which to function.

It is clear that although Spanish dancing in the past was constantly subjected to outside influences, it always succeeded in maintaining its own individuality. The traditional dancing of the country has survived the test of time by adhering to fundamentally Spanish standards. Whether this state of affairs will continue remains to be seen. Only the future can reveal whether the dancing Spaniards are prepared to go on building upon their own tradition —accepting the controls that go with it—or decide to branch out and imitate a European style of classical ballet, copying the free movement fashionable at the moment and accepted by ballet audiences throughout the world.

The modern trend of ballet does not always satisfy dance critics who feel that a new impulse in keeping with modern life is needed, but they do not seem to know where this is to come from, nor how it is to be brought about. Spain, with her superb dance tradition, could well become the forcing ground for just such a new movement, since the prospect of a Spanish ballet in the near future, is brighter than it has been for a long time. The establishment of a new theatre with a permanent company backed by the government, presenting (it may be hoped) a succession of ballet creations each season, produced under the most up-to-date conditions, achieved by the young artists, dancers, musicians and scenic designers with a fresh outlook, might easily prove to be the impetus required to bring about the eagerly awaited renaissance in ballet production, for which the world is waiting.

Ballet in Spain has always had a struggle to survive and, looking through her history, it seems as though it takes a hundred years before public interest is sufficiently aroused to make any attempt to repair the damage done during the previous century. The loss of the Teatro Real, demolished and not yet replaced, was a calamity but, nevertheless, it still represents a milestone in the balletic achievement of Spain. Thanks to the efforts of leading Spanish dance artists, a nucleus of young dancers exists, sufficiently experienced to enter the portals of the national theatre-to-be. That is where the future growth of Spanish ballet will have to be concentrated. These young people will be taking up the threads of past fulfilment to weave them into the pattern of a neo-Spanish ballet which, in time, may come to be part of the fabric of Spanish life.

There will be many changes but signs of future development are already apparent; the only element missing is the theatre. As soon as that is supplied, there will be no lack of talent, enthusiasm and vitality forthcoming for, as everybody knows, dancing is inherent in the Spanish people. Have they not a refrain which tells us that every Spaniard comes into this world, dancing?

The Past

A SATISFACTORY answer to any inquiry into the state of dancing today in Spain may only be found by delving into the past and comparing conditions then with now. This also applies even to the simplest questions. There are two in particular that seem to fascinate Spanish dance lovers—if one may judge by the times they are asked—and these are: 'When did the Spaniards first start to play the castanets?' and 'When did they start to dance?'

Spanish dancers, when interrogated are usually at a loss for an answer—they have probably never given the matter even a thought. On one occasion, in my presence that great artist Antonio looked ingenuously at the enquirer and, turning to me, said: 'You are interested in dance history. Do you know? I don't.' At the time neither did I and this made me decide to look into the matter.

Briefly, the picture that emerged indicated that the pattern of Spanish dancing followed along the same lines as that of other countries in primitive times. That is to say, dancing was used on religious occasions, or to celebrate victories in battle or, simply, as a means of recreation. The dances of the Peninsula varied from region to region, according to the race, language and religion of the people living in them. The inhabitants of the Iberian Peninsula were distinguished by their diverse customs, habits and dress. Those from one region might have nothing in common with their neighbours in the adjoining one.

In the early days, the country was divided into kingdoms and each had an independent ruler. Pride of race and region was very pronounced and, as if to impress upon the others how infinitely superior their way of life was, the people passed the time attacking one another. Continuous sparring went on until the end of the fifteenth century when finally the country settled down and became one united nation.

In addition to these internal squabbles that kept the inhabitants busy, there were also others on a grander scale, when alien armies attacked them. Spain has always attracted foreigners, many of whom went with the sole idea of conquering the land and settling there. The presence of these intruders considerably affected the social life of the country, and in time constant foreign interchange influenced all the people's activities.

In order to visualize how Spanish dancing developed in the way it did, these facts must be borne in mind and, at the same time, it might be useful to give a brief outline of the general pattern of life during the undocumented period. That is, from prehistoric times to the Fall of the Roman Empire in the fifth century, when the country was overrun by diverse alien forces, until she was finally dominated by the Visigoths who remained in power until the eighth century. The Moors came next and occupied the Peninsula for nearly seven hundred years. Only after their departure was the country welded into a national entity. This process was hastened in 1497, by the marriage of Ferdinand and Isabella, when the Crowns of Leon and Castille were finally united.

Doubtless, because the Iberian Peninsula was in an incessant state of warfare for so long, much valuable material in the way of documentation has been lost, dispersed or destroyed. This is why at present so little is known about the roots of Spanish dancing during the early days of its growth. General references appear from time to time, in musical and historical works and it is these we have to rely upon for information. If, by any chance, any pre-medieval treatises on dancing existed, they do not appear to have survived and it was not until the Middle Ages that it became possible to observe the shape that Spanish dancing might take.

The founders of the Spanish race were the Celts and the hypothetical Iberians who, together, formed a race called Celtiberians, by which name it has been known since the third century B.C. The dances then in existence were chiefly of a religious or military nature, although the Iberian women were known to be fond of dancing as a means of recreation. Other groups of people were inhabiting the Peninsula at the same time and pictorial evidence suggests that they all danced. Designs on excavated vases of Iberian origin, and those of neolithic times found in primitive cave drawings, show the positions the dancers used, how they were grouped and the kind of clothing they wore (pls. 1–4). Strabo alluded to the Celtiberians living in the central part of Spain, dancing at the time of the full moon; while in the south, the men and women of Bastetania linked hands to dance. In the north, the Montaneses danced to the sound of flute and trumpet and this is probably the earliest reference to the type of instrument used to accompany dancing. Strabo described dancers leaping into the air or squatting on their heels, bending the body forward—which sounds uncommonly like steps now associated with Russian dancing, and which are very prevalent today in Galician dancing in North-West Spain.[1]

Seeking trade, fortune, or both, many races settled in the Peninsula and the newcomers all contributed something to the growth of the nation and to her dancing. The Phoenicians were among the first arrivals and the Hebrews followed shortly after them. The exact date of their coming is unknown but their entry into the country is of the utmost importance when considering the elements that have gone into development of Spanish dancing. Sacred dancing was a feature of their religious life then and today, Spain is perhaps the only remaining land in Europe where dancing still takes place in church.

About 600 B.C. the Greeks penetrated the country and settled in the south and on the south-east coast. Hellenic culture profoundly influenced the life of the people living in the Peninsula. The part dancing played in the ancient Greek civilization is too well known to require elaboration here. The Romans came after the Greeks and remained to dominate the country from 215 B.C. to A.D. 409. During that period they latinized the lives of the people by introducing Roman customs, language, thermal establishments, horse and chariot races, gladiatorial contests, bullfights and magnificent

[1]Estrabon: *Geografia*, vol. 3, p. 155. Madrid 1734.

theatrical spectacles. They built roads, bridges, aqueducts and fine theatres.

The Roman were known for their love of spectacular entertainments on a vast scale, including tragic and comic plays in which dancing and mimed movements played an important part. Relics of open-air Roman circuses and amphitheatres are scattered about Spain today, bearing testimony to the popularity of these productions. Dancing as light entertainment formed part of the celebrated Roman feasts and there the native dancers of the Peninsula had abundant opportunity to show off their dances. On a more modest scale, the same type of dancing took place in taverns much as it does today in similar haunts. The venerable antiquity of Spanish dancing is equalled perhaps only by that of the vine. Allusions to dancing in Roman times give the impression that the Roman occupants of the country we now call Spain were not particularly interested in dancing themselves but preferred to act as spectators and let the Hispanic dancers entertain them. Yet, while admiring their dancing, some of the poets, philosophers and historians at least, found something in them to carp about and that was usually the gyrations of the dancers' hips. Various epithets of the 'provocative', 'lascivious' and 'obscene' order were applied to their dances. Martial damned with faint praise the sinuous movements which he liked but found 'lecherous'.[2] Juvenal proclaimed that he could never permit such dancing displays in his humble abode.[3]

This is all very interesting but it might have been more enlightening had these gentlemen criticized less and given more precise details as to the form of the dance or any indication of the steps they found so disturbing. Dark hints were dropped occasionally that the dancing maidens were drunk and then the usual observations about swaying movements were made. It would appear from this that it was the manner of dancing rather than the dances themselves that seduced certain members of the audience while, at the same time, shocking them. This sort of reaction is worth noting, for it has persisted right through the ages and may still be observed today. Spanish dancing is curious in that it engenders a mixture of

[2]Martial: *Epigramas* v. lxxviii.
[3]Juvenal: *Satire* xl. 162–75.

admiration and censure among many who watch it. Very much later, in the sixteenth century, these disturbing hip movements caused two dances to be officially banned—this applied particularly to the chaconne and sarabande. Constant vigilance, severe punishment and everlasting criticism from official quarters has done nothing to eliminate these much publicized movements and they are still typical of many Spanish dances in various parts of Spain. Tell any Spanish dancer nowadays that she has 'honey in her hips' and she will be highly flattered. The dual process of admiration and condemnation continues and by now is all part of Spanish dance tradition.

In Hispano-Roman times, danced interludes were quite fashionable between the courses at the notorious Roman feasts, famous for their opulence and the levity of the assembled company. They were designed first and foremost to entertain the Romans and their guests. Not a great deal is known about these dances; presumably they adhered to some form but we do not know what it was. We do know that the dancers made a lot of noise with 'crotalos' when they danced, which may have been the forerunners of castanets. They apparently served the same purpose—to mark the rhythm of the dance, accentuate the dancers' movements and irritate people with sensitive hearing. The noise they made appealed to some, others condemned it. Noisy though they were, we are not told from what they were made, but they must have been fashioned from some material light enough for a girl to handle easily—possibly nacre or some other shell like castanets, for oyster and similar shells had long been used by the inhabitants of the Mediterranean coast to accompany their dances. The din referred to was not made by the girls dancing, but by the crotalo accompaniment. The chief interest centred on the feminine aspect of Hispanic dancing in those days, or so it seems. There is no evidence to show that the male dancers made the sort of impact upon the audiences then, as they do nowadays.

Perhaps the most striking feature about this period was the fact that the Romans never seemed inclined to interfere with the indigenous dancing they found in the Peninsula. This is remarkable when it is remembered that in most things the people had been obliged to adopt Roman customs. It was no mean achievement that the Iberian inhabitants maintained independence in their dancing when they had lost it in most other fields of human endeavour and were able, even encouraged, to continue dancing in their own way. Far from suppressing the dancing of the Iberians, the Romans sponsored it. The first impresario on record may well have been the man sent by a senator from Rome to recruit hundreds of dancing girls from the Peninsula to bring to the metropolis. Those early Hispanic dance influences spread far beyond the confines of the Peninsula. These conditions lasted throughout the Roman occupation but the picture changed after A.D. 476, however, when others came to replace the Romans and occupy the land.

DANCING UNDER THE VISIGOTHS

Alans, Swabians, Vandals and Visigoths poured into Spain from the north. Wave after wave of Gothic hordes spread through the country. Finally, in the sixth century the Visigoths triumphed, settled in the Peninsula and made Toledo their capital. These aggressive, warmongering people were more interested in the art of war than any other. During the early days of their occupation, all their energies were directed towards establishing themselves; they had little time for dancing, learning, and still less for the art of living. The Hispano-Romans regarded them as savages not only because they dressed in animal skins and wore their hair long but mainly on account of their being Aryan and heretics. Christianity was part of Hispano-Roman life and had been ever since the first century A.D. Since the Visigoths were not orthodox Christians, the inhabitants of the Peninsula could not consider them akin to anything other than interlopers. No reform was possible until the races began to exchange ideas. At first, the conquerors tried unsuccessfully to impose their crude manners upon the Hispano-Romans who, in turn, reversed the process and succeeded in modifying the invaders' coarseness. Visigothic education aimed at forming warriors and manly, warlike games were encouraged; these became the forerunners of the medieval tournaments. Thermal establishments with their gymnasia did not interest the Visigoths in the least and they

The Past

lost no time in closing them down. The grandiose public performances so beloved of the Romans were likewise dispensed with. That
essential part of Hispano-Roman life, the habit of theatre-going,
came to an abrupt end, as elaborate theatrical productions played
absolutely no part in the Visigothic conception of life. As the
process of reorganizing the country went on, there were no funds
available for what were considered to be pleasurable luxuries
and, furthermore, there were no audiences to support big theatres.
Taste in entertainment changed as it did in so many other things.
Functions became more intimate, on a smaller scale altogether, but
dancing was still associated with banquets, feasting and revelry.
These were held in connection with private domestic events such as
weddings and family reunions, and there were also receptions held in
honour of distinguished civic or military visitors. Dancing girls did
not figure in these for they were replaced by male dancers and
mimes, whose crude performances were notorious for their grossness. This appeared to be the Visigothic idea of good entertainment.

The name given to these artists was 'mimico' or 'histrione' and,
according to the definition of the words by the seventh-century
scholar, Bishop Isidore of Seville,[4] 'histriones' were 'men dressing
as women, making impure gestures as they recalled past events and
told their stories in movement'. 'Mimicos' were so called 'because
they portrayed human beings'.

The author would tell his story and the mimico would then
interpret it in movement. The tale was composed in such a manner
that it could be adapted to the movements of the mimico's body.

The taste for classical comedy and heroic tragedy declined as the
fashion for mimicos and histriones gained ground. These were
replaced by pantomimes and plays in which the artists dressed
themselves up, made lewd gestures, sang obscene songs and
performed dances of a similar nature. Entertainment under the
Visigothic régime was in deplorably bad taste. It was little else than
a public exhibition of vulgarity and at times fell to the lowest level
of farce. Licentiousness was not only confined to the mime and
dancing of the histriones and mimicos; it extended to popular
dancing in which both sexes participated. At one point, it reached

[4]St. Isidore of Seville: *Etymologia*.

31

such a state of wild abandon that the Church authorities intervened and forbade men and women from dancing together in public.[5] Nor were they allowed to wear masks of any kind. Men might not dress as women, nor women as men. Dances connected with the wine harvest were considered to be especially pernicious and condemned on the grounds that they were too closely connected with paganism and were therefore unhealthy and morally harmful to the faithful.

As time went by, the Visigoths gradually developed a taste for the pleasant social customs they found in the Peninsula, introduced there by the Romans. They began to wear Roman dress, the women adorned themselves with jewellery in the Roman manner and used scent. Yet, while basking in the luxury of the newly discovered accoutrements of Latin civilization in Hispano-Roman life, they were at heart fundamentally Germanic. Real integration with the inhabitants of the country only came about when they finally became orthodox Catholics. The Catholicism of Rome became the recognized religion of the land towards the end of the sixth century—not that this put an end to the perpetual bickering that went on among the Visigothic nobles, nor mitigated the violence of their methods when imposing their beliefs upon the unbaptized. It was apparent that they were absolutely determined to stamp out everything pertaining to their former paganism. Up to that time, the Jews had always lived, worked and prospered in the Peninsula without any hindrance from their fellow men, but after the Visigoths were converted they became so fanatically intolerant that many Jews allowed themselves to be baptized into the new faith out of sheer desperation. This was not enough to satisfy the bellicose Visigoths who were quite resolved to subjugate the entire land. Persecuting all who opposed them, they forged ahead, imposing their will upon all the inhabitants, with the most fearful ruthlessness. A period of unrest and confusion ensued, further complicated by dissension among the nobles that arose through their jockeying for power. The chief victims of their intolerance were the Jews, many of whom were powerful and wealthy. They were declared to be slaves, deprived of their wealth and forbidden to practise their religion.

[5]Concilia Trullanum (A.D. 602), Canon 62.

Those who could, fled the country and sought refuge in North Africa.

Towards the end of the seventh century, the Arabs were planning to invade the Peninsula from North Africa and, profiting by the internal discord then prevailing, helped by the Jews, they overran the country. They occupied it within the space of a few years, with the exception of the north, where the Basques and Asturians successfully maintained their independence. The northerners thus became the custodians of national art and this is probably why it is generally considered that the oldest and purest form of Spanish dancing seen today comes from the north.

The Arabs refrained from imposing their religion upon the Christians during the early days of their occupation of the Peninsula. Indeed they despised them so much that they would not allow them to ride anything so superior as an Arab horse, nor wear Arab dress. Jews were protected by the caliphate, in return for the aid they had rendered. They were even allotted their own part of the towns known as the 'Juderia' where they were free to live in peace and practise their own religion. The Moorish section of the town was known as the 'Morería'. Christians were tolerated, but they had to curtail certain religious customs such as bell-ringing and do nothing to annoy their new masters. Some Christians were converted to Islam—not out of conviction, but usually from necessity or ambition. In this rich mosaic of humanity consisting of Greek, Roman, Jewish, and now Arabic, elements, the arts began to flourish anew. As far as dancing was concerned, it had survived despite the rigorous censorship the Visigoths had imposed upon it. A most fecund period in the development of Spanish dance was at hand.

UNDER THE MOSLEMS

The Arabs liked dancing girls but, unlike the Romans, brought their own with them. Not all of these were professional; some dancers were imported as slaves—male and female—and were obliged to dance when required. The professional dancers coming from the East were engaged by the caliphates, were well paid, and became so immensely popular that they became fashionable at the Christian courts in the north. Little was heard about the national dancing of the people but it may be assumed that the unconquered continued dancing in their own way and some time would have to elapse before they were influenced by new oriental movements and rhythms.

References to Moorish dances in the Iberian Peninsula at that time were confined to literary allusions which were tiresomely vague. There is not a shred of pictorial evidence available, for the Moslem religion forbade its followers to portray the human form in works of art. There are no pictures to give any clues concerning the postures, groupings or positions of the dancers. Music fares a little better since musicologists have investigated the musical forms then introduced from the Orient. Rhythmically, dance form follows musical form and the findings of these historians are useful in suggesting the rhythmic pattern and construction that might later shape the dances. They are helpful but not conclusive, because they are very much divided in their opinions on the subject. The streams of influence involved in Hispanic music appear to have been those of the Celts, the Jews and the Arabs, but nobody appears to be very sure which of these predominated. Investigations revealed that liturgical music was already highly developed when the Moors first arrived, and by the time they finally settled in the Peninsula their music was profoundly influenced by that already existing there—of the Hebrews. It does not follow from this that because Arabic music became so prominent and better known than Celtic music that it was more important. Moreover, there were strong Celtic influences in the Peninsula and it was Celtic music, after all, that determined the birth of European music. That much was known about musical influences, but we cannot be so sure about those in dancing. It may be presumed that the situation was similar but since no parallel research has been carried out in the realm of Hispanic dancing the subject at present remains shrouded in a cloak of hypothesis.

Quite the most brilliant court existing in the eighth century was that at Cordova. Foremost among the pastimes was dancing. It was held in high esteem as a princely accomplishment and considered

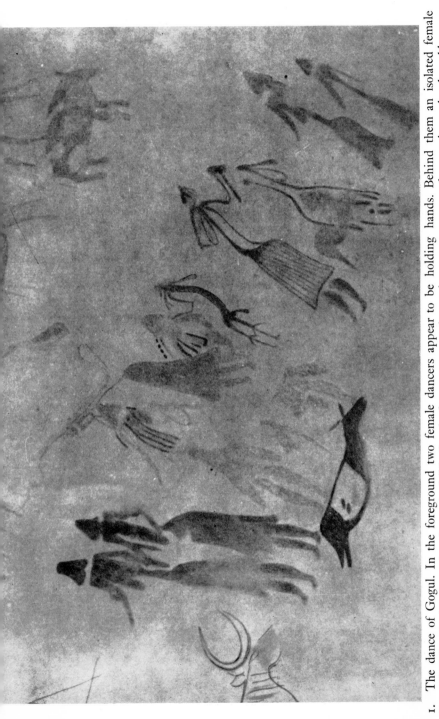

1. The dance of Gogul. In the foreground two female dancers appear to be holding hands. Behind them an isolated female figure has her back to us. An almost invisible female figure near to the nude man appears to be wearing a bead necklace or rosary. Two more pairs of women are to the right of the male phallic figure.

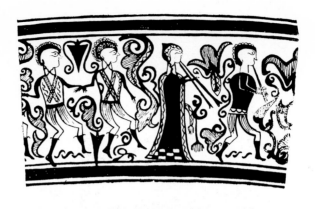

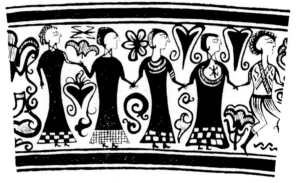

2. Vase design of men and women dancing.

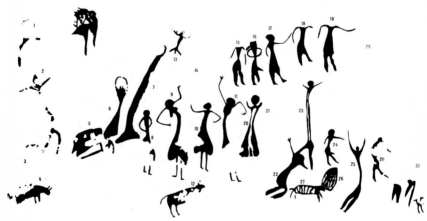

3. A phallic dance as at Gogul showing characteristic dance poses. Several of the figures have their arms raised above the head. Figure 10 has her right arm curved in front of the body while her left is arched over the head, similar to the position used today in Andalusian dances. Figure 16 is a man with an uncommonly large phallus; in Bronze Age times this was a typical representation. On the right side of the frieze three women are with four men. From the 'Barranco de los Grajos' (Murcia).

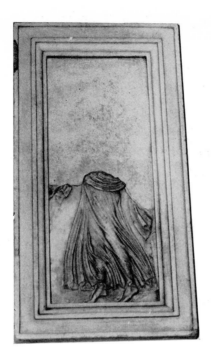

4. Roman remains found in Evora (Lusitania). Note rising ball of the foot.

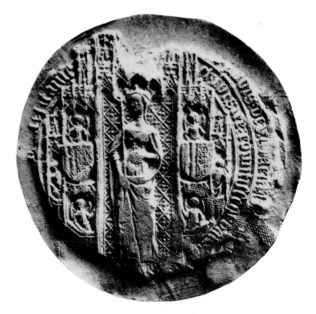

5. Relief sculpture of Violant de Bar giving an impression of the weight of the costume of that period.

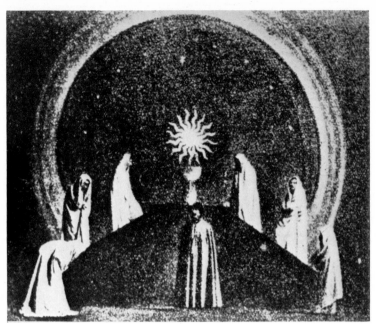

6. Sixteenth century mystery play with balletic grouping.

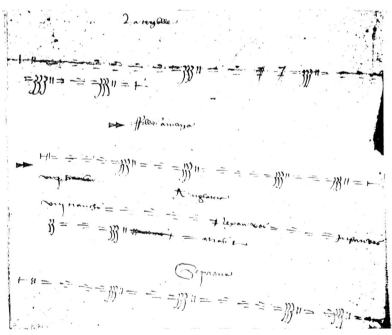

7. Detail from Lerida Manuscript (Spain) 1496. Note difference in the type of notation between this and the Salisbury Manuscript (opposite). *Filles a Marier* in the centre

8. Detail of the Salisbury Manuscript (1497) showing *Filles a Marier* at the top.

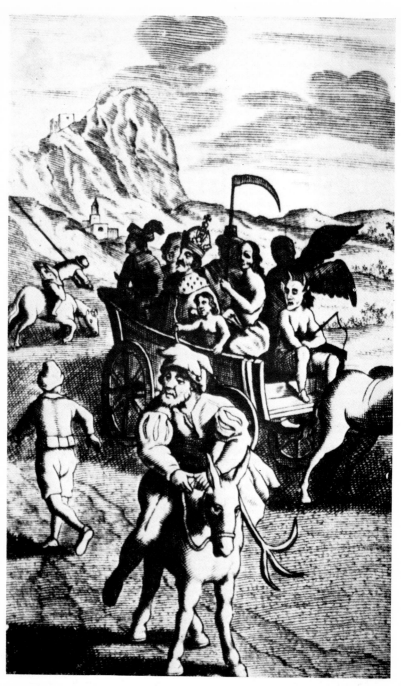

9. Wandering players who travelled through the villages of Castille in the sixteenth and seventeenth centuries.

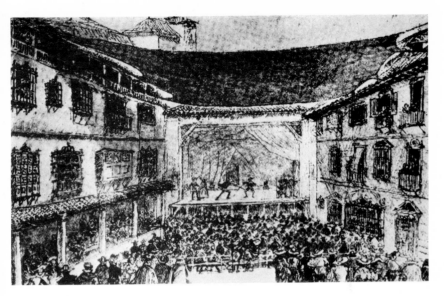

10. Reconstruction of the Corral del Principe *c.* 1660.

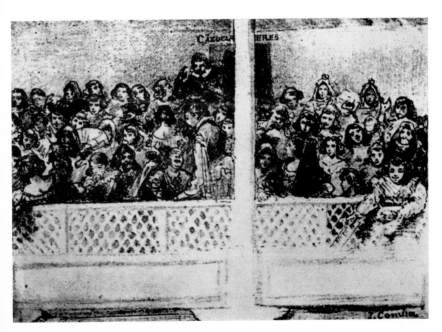

11. The ladies' pit (La Cazuela) at Corral del Principe; seventeenth century.

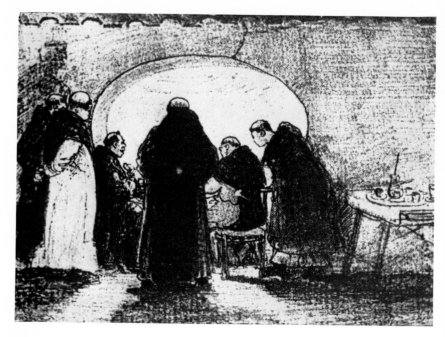

12. The scholars' box.

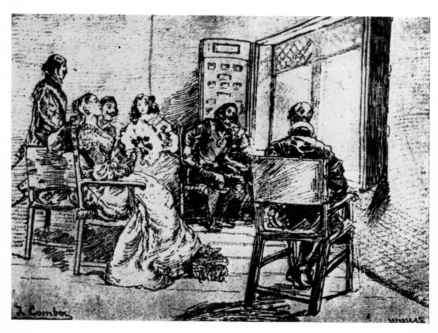

13. Box for nobility; seventeenth century.

to be part of every cultivated young person's education. Even the highest dignitaries were not above disporting themselves at banquets and similar functions. In addition to this social aspect of dancing was the most spectacular kind found in the solos of exhibition dancing given by dancers especially engaged for that purpose. As far as one can see, nearly all the dancing was connected with convivial occasions at the Cordovese caliphate and, surprisingly, with wine bibbing; this, in spite of the fact that the consumption of alcoholic liquor was sternly forbidden by Moslem law. The drinking of wine in Andalusia was quite common among all inhabitants, whether Moslems, Jews or Christians; it inspired Moslem poets to write odes in praise of the golden Andalusian wines. Obviously there was nothing heavy, tedious, or austere about life at the caliphate and dancing there was of a quite different quality from the sedate measures then currently performed at the Christian courts of the same period.

Once established, the pattern of life at the Moorish courts appeared to be one of gay sensuality and the social dancing has to be set against this background. It was all in complete contrast with the austerity of the former Visigothic régime where social dancing had no chance to flourish. It now seemed possible for new ground to be prepared in which once more dancing could continue to grow. Life changed for many people; distinguished Christian nobles, Jewish scholars and Arab dignitaries were all received and entertained at the caliphate. The effect of oriental influence made itself felt in all branches of the fine arts and in science and learning generally. In the Hispanic world of art and entertainment fashions were gradually modified as these influences penetrated the Christian world, entering all spheres of life, and these changes were particularly visible in the aristocratic world.

At the commencement of the ninth century, Cordova was not only a centre of learning and artistic activity but also represented all that was civilized in life at that time. One of the great innovators was a musician. In A.D. 821 he was brought from Persia to play and sing to the sultan who happened to be a great music-lover. Soon he became the court favourite, not only on account of his musical gifts, but also because he was an outstanding personality. Known as The

Blackbird, his real name was Zyriab, and apart from his music he added much to the comfort and amenities of daily life. The women were overjoyed when he opened a ninth-century equivalent of a beauty parlour where, if they wished, they could have their hair trimmed in a fringe, then considered a great novelty; or have their eyebrows plucked and faces made up. He revolutionized feminine fashions, introducing dark colours and heavy fabrics for the winter season and pastel shades and light materials for the summer. In addition to these exploits, he ventured into the culinary domain and initiated the court into the mystery of working out a well-balanced menu. No longer was it in fashion to heap all one's food together on one plate. A meal had to commence with soup, followed by a meat dish seasoned, so we are told, 'in the Baghdad manner', and it concluded with succulent sweet dishes made from nuts and honey, or fruit paste stuffed with almond or pistachio nuts. Fine food led to other refinements and Zyriab was responsible for introducing tooth paste to the inhabitants. Professionally, he was known to be something of an inventor. Up to his day, lutes generally had possessed only four strings, but he accompanied himself when he sang on a five-stringed lute which he plucked with a plectrum made from an eagle's quill.

This easy tenor of life endured until the early eleventh century. The Moors had ruled progressively and well during this first occupation. Moorish soldiers had intermarried with local inhabitants and marriage between Moorish and Christian noble families also took place. In A.D. 1032, the caliphate of Cordova fell. Tribes from Jordan poured in, to settle and remain in the Peninsula until 1146. Today, Spaniards appear to use the words 'Moors' and 'Arabs' indiscriminately which is puzzling for foreigners. Each invasion, in fact, brought in tribes from Persia, Syria and Africa and this constant fusion of races exerted considerable influence upon the physique, language, and, inevitably, the dancing of the country. The dances of southern Spain today reflect influences from the Orient—noticeably so, in the use of the arms and wrists, upper part of the body and also in some of the complex un-occidental rhythms.

After the fall of Cordova, the centre of interest moved to Seville where life became merrier and more convivial than ever. Regattas and aquatic festivals were added to the other well established forms of open air parties. A favourite diversion known as a 'zambra', where men, women and slaves sang and danced until dawn, set a new style in entertainment. Moors, Jews and Christians fraternized and the local wine flowed freely. Teeming with poetic allusions to the beauty of the surroundings, chronicles of the time describe fine concerts of music which were given as an adjunct to the magnificent receptions for which, by then, the Peninsula was famous, Seville being one of the leading centres of musical culture in the world.

Nocturnal open-air parties continued to be highly favoured and delighted the local inhabitants, whose enthusiasm was not shared by foreign visitors when they found their slumbers disturbed by the noise. Slave-girls sang and danced to the accompaniment of drums and lutes, so we are told but not a great deal is known about the nature of their dances. Also, it is not always clear whether all these entertainers came from the Orient, or if some local talent was also employed. It is not difficult to imagine in the hot, still Andalusian nights, the din made by beating drums, trilling pipes and wailing eastern laments mingling with the applause, laughter and chatter from the enthusiastic audiences. Many of the parties were of modest dimensions and were held in the patios or gardens of the houses. A Moorish visitor once heard such exquisite music in the night that he thought he must be dreaming. He rose from his bed to investigate and beheld a neighbouring garden, where only about twenty people were gathered, partaking of liqueurs, sweetmeats and fruit spread out before them. As they savoured these delicacies, a slave from Baghdad sang sweetly, accompanying herself most beautifully upon the lute.

How different was this gentle refined pattern of living from that of the previous Nordic occupants of the land! The Arabs knew so well how to adapt themselves to the lovely climate of the southern part of the Peninsula, making the most of the natural resources of the country and adding to them, by growing flowering shrubs, trees and plants that they took the trouble to bring with them from the East. They revived the cult of water, not only in baths indoors, but outdoors as well, in decorative lakes and pools, or tinkling fountains which adorned the courtyards then and remain to this day, so typical of Andalusian patios. In this pleasant setting, music, dance and song flourished.

As the Moors obtained an ever firmer foothold, oriental influences continued to seep into the fabric of life. Social dancing was indulged in by the Moors during the early days of the occupation but there is no evidence to suggest that mixed social dancing was encouraged among the other inhabitants. This came later. The main stream of influence appears to have flowed through the exotic dances performed, either by well-paid professionals, or slaves whose dances at times were considered to be in such dubious taste that it was the cause of adverse criticism. This is all very reminiscent of the past and so was the reaction. Far from curtailing interest, it had the opposite effect and the time came when Moorish entertainers were so highly thought of that they began to be attached to the Christian courts as well. In this way Moorish art penetrated aristocratic life throughout the land.

In the Middle Ages, it was quite customary to find the troubadours installed at court side by side with professional Moorish artists. It has been suggested that it was in this way that the troubadours discovered and succumbed to the influences from the East. Certainly the Moorish artists set a style in the Christian courts which the troubadours followed. Fascinated by new and unfamiliar songs and dances, troubadours and minstrels did not hesitate to adopt the novel tunes and rhythms which they elaborated later. The dances performed by these artists were at that time accompanied by songs, musical instruments or both. The difference between these two distinct grades of artists should here be noted. Troubadours were honoured guests at court, frequently they rose to positions of power, such a one was Mossen Borra whose tomb may be found in the crypt of Barcelona Cathedral. He was a linguist, treated royalty as equals, addressing them as 'dear cousin' and, indeed, was entrusted with diplomatic missions. Some people thought he was a spy. The troubadours could and did earn huge fortunes, unlike the poor wandering minstrels, who were at the other end of the social scale in the world of entertainment. The troubadours in the Peninsula formed an élite, comparable with the highly esteemed professionals brought from the East, while the minstrels were akin to the slave entertainers, except that they were not attached to one house, but wandered from place to place, poor, servile, dependent upon the charity of those who watched them sing, play or dance.

In the early twelfth century when the Cordovese Caliphate fell, dancing in the south was slowly evolving into an art form composite of elements from the East and the West, resulting from the exchange of reciprocal influences which had been going on continuously from the eighth century. It was only in the north that these influences took longer to penetrate and become incorporated into the local dances. The northerners were cut off from the southerners because, like the Scots and the Welsh in the British Isles, they had sought refuge behind the mountains and thus escaped conquest. Their dancing remained the indigenous folk-dancing of the country. This was particularly true of the dances from the Basque country, Galicia in north-western Spain, and the Asturias. The inhabitants of those lands had most successfully shut themselves away from external interference.

Between the eleventh and twelfth centuries things began to change in the north. While the Moors had been busy establishing themselves in the south, the Christians in the rest of the land had not for one moment relinquished their efforts to reclaim their country. Slowly extending their territory, they spread towards the centre, until they reached Castille. To help them achieve their ends, foreign mercenaries from all parts of Europe came in to assist with the task and it was thus that European influences penetrated the northern part of the country. The dance influences were predominantly French.

THE RECONQUEST

At that period, the country was still divided into kingdoms and France, as a good and close neighbour, obligingly provided the kings with consorts. The second wife of Alfonso VI was French: Dulcie, Countess of Provence, married Berenguer II,[6] and it was during their reign that Aragon and Barcelona were united. The provinces

[6]Ramon Berenguer (1096–1131).

today known as Catalonia and Aragon were in this way linked with Provence. French court dancing began to permeate that of the Peninsula. To complicate the matter further, diverse elements more difficult to define, due to the ever increasing intermingling of races and people as the reconquest of the country progressed, began to creep in. As the rulers of Leon, Galicia and the Asturias pressed on from the north, gradually extending their hold upon the country, the reclaimed cities had to be repopulated—chiefly by Christians and Mozarabes, who were those Christians who had been forced to work for the Moslems. This close contact with Moslems had heavily influenced their work, particularly noticeable in their arts and crafts. After the Moors had been driven out of Toledo and the new conquerors reached Castille, the ancient Visigothic capital became the seat of Hispanic nationalism, and centre of European influence, and once more Toledo rose supreme, the capital city.

The fact that the sole preoccupation of the Christians had been to reclaim the land for themselves, meant that all their energies had to be directed towards this goal and, therefore, the pursuit of the liberal professions and the arts had been left in the hands of the Jews and Moslems. Consequently, these influences predominated for some time, that is, until the French came on the scene. The Christian inhabitants of the Peninsula had received powerful support from the House of Burgundy in their struggle to expel the Moors.[7] This event happened at a time when dance form was beginning to be developed in France. This subject will be dealt with at greater length in the next chapter. Suffice to mention here that dances then adhered to set rules concerning figures, steps and phrasing of movements. The dances the French brought with them were added to those they found in the new capital. Dancing in the centre of the Peninsula flourished anew, consisting of native Castilian elements with oriental influences superimposed upon them and very soon new steps and a foreign style were added to this composite base.

Quite familiar with Moorish customs, the new sovereigns were profoundly impressed by the sumptuous luxury of the sultan's courts and did their best to copy them. They continued to employ

[7]Conquest of Toledo: 1085.

Moorish dancers, singers and musicians. Alfonso the Wise (1253–84) was a great patron of Moorish art and patiently collected many of the vocal and instrumental works in the repertoire of the professional Moorish musicians at court. Some of these pieces were dance tunes. The Spanish musicologist, Don Julian Ribera, considered them to be a curious and admirable example of the musical culture prevalent in the peninsula during the Middle Ages. What is of particular interest to dancers are the dance tunes from diverse regions that are still used today. Another curiosity is to find exmples of 'canto hondo', or deep song, in this thirteenth-century collection. These are generally associated nowadays with gypsy singing and dancing, commonly known as 'flamenco', but the gypsies had not yet set foot in the Peninsula! There were some charming court dance melodies and it is clear from this that in the medieval period the inhabitants were perfectly familiar with these three aspects of dancing.[8]

Throughout this period, dancing was disseminated in a variety of ways. Popular dances were not written down but passed on from one generation to another. People began to enjoy more free time than they had ever dreamed of in the past and, to amuse themselves they devised new means of entertainment. Simple scenic plays in which dancing played a prominent part were produced. Those taking part in them were amateurs, who tended to look down on the few professionals who helped them out and earned their living by acting and dancing. Folk-dancing became most popular, the dances were infinitely varied, depending upon the region from which they came and were usually performed in the open air. Competitions were held between neighbouring districts and this is where the strong regional influences that characterize Spanish dancing today will have to be sought. As for the gentry, they learned their dances from the wandering dancing masters who went from castle to castle instructing the nobles in the latest dances from home and abroad. In short, dancing became a pleasant pastime for all and sundry, whether they were native inhabitants, visitors or pilgrims, of whom there were vast quantities. A profitable exchange of ideas and

[8]Selected from *Las Cantigas de Alfonso el Sabio* by Julian Ribera. (A short list of dance tunes may be found at end of book in Appendix A.)

customs resulted, which directly influenced the indigenous dancing of the country.

The simple dances of the people were taken and used profusely in the thirteenth-century mystery plays. In this way they were transformed from a straightforward, natural dance form into a spectacular one. It was a perfect way of bringing them to the notice of the masses and making them more aware of their own type of dancing. Sacred dances were a salient feature of these religious manifestations. A specimen of this kind of play, which is quite unique today, may still be seen at Elche near Alicante. It takes place on the evenings of 14 and 15 August. The *Mystery of Elche* is semi-religious, semi-lyrical in character, set to music of the thirteenth century and performed with traditional ritual in St. Mary's church. The theme deals with the Mystery of the Assumption of the Holy Mother into heaven. Stage effects are produced by means of the original primitive machinery, which still works. Clouds part in the dome of the church, and an angel descends in a ball of fire, as though from heaven. A choral arrangement of the thirteenth-century music was rearranged in the sixteenth century and this is what is used today. The artists taking part in the play are not professional, but follow the ancient custom—they are drawn from the ranks of the ordinary citizens of Elche.

All social dancing had to be set against the extraordinarily rich pattern of life that was established in the Iberian Peninsula during those stirring times: the contrast presented between the restraining influence of the Christians, alongside the carefree sensuality of the Moorish occupants should be noted. Quite early in the thirteenth century, there were more upheavals in the south. This time, the focal point of culture shifted to Granada. The splendour of life in the kingdom of Granada surpassed anything previously known.[9] The apex of Moorish civilization had been reached, for already the end of Moslem domination was in sight. Learning was protected by the sultan and, with the foundation of the university, attained its full glory. The Moors were very absorbed by the art of living in all its plenitude and the cultivation of the arts and learning was most important to them. Entertainments of all kinds—zambras,

[9]Moorish kingdom of Granada founded in 1238.

The Past

firework displays, feasting and games were outstanding elements of social life at court. Young nobles with delightful-sounding oriental names practised their dancing, along with other gentlemanly pursuits like horsemanship, music and singing, then considered part of the necessary equipment for the life of any young person of noble birth. Lovely little princesses danced 'extremadamente' and played music in the Castillian and Moorish manner—apparently the two most important styles of performance then current.

At that time a little more information was given about the social dancing that took place. The first Moorish king of Granada commanded that the guests should dance after the banquet given in honour of the leading citizens. On the occasion of a zambra given in connection with wedding festivities attended by the king and queen, specific allusions were made to the dancing that took place then. After the ceremony, they returned to the Alhambra with the young couple and a royal banquet took place on the same evening. The newly-married bride and bridegroom led the dancing; the king partnered the queen and they, it seemed, 'danced very well together'. We are left wondering what the dance was they did so well together, but we are not told. Exhibition dancing fares somewhat better. A good idea of the quality of the professional dancers so commonly employed to divert the guests in Moorish Spain may be obtained from the following quotation. We are indebted to Don Emilio Garcia Gomez for his translation of a book of poems by Ibn Said al-Magribi. The title of the poem is 'The Dancer'.[10]

THE DANCER

With his varying movements he plays with the heart
and is robed with charm when denuded of clothing,

swaying as a branch in its garden
playing as a gazelle in its lair

Darting backwards and forwards his movements play with the
intelligence of the onlookers

much as fortune plays at will with men
touching his head with his feet like a well tempered sword
that can be bent until the point touches the hilt.

[10]Emilio Garcia Gomez: *Poemas arabigo-andaluces* (3rd edition Madrid—Buenos Aires 1943). Coleccion Austral, Espasa Calpe No. 162. Number 71.)

43

The same author was so inspired by the performance of a tightrope dancer that he described him soaring into the air like a bird, only transformed into man as he descended from space to stand on the wire, quivering like a lance and twisting like a snake.[11]

How useful it would have been had social dances of the period been treated with such poetic imagery and vision, but they are only mentioned by name. Frequent allusions were made to the zambra, alleged to be the 'most famous and artistic dance in the whole of the Peninsula', but we are left to guess why. We are at least told that the dancers were 'holding hands as is customary in this dance' and that is all. The zambra was often used in religious processions but it seems highly unlikely that holding hands between dancers of both sexes would be encouraged in a dance in a religious context in those days. The word 'zambra', of Arabic origin, referred not only to a dance, but could also be applied to a band of musicians, or a nocturnal gathering; obviously some sort of revelry took place at these parties for that kind of zambra was soon abolished once the Catholic kings came to the throne.

Unlike their predecessors, the Moors did not object to the public dancing in the streets. Indeed they encouraged it. A royal proclamation was made and sent out to all the Morerias in the kingdom, demanding all who knew how, to come out and dance the folias to welcome a visiting prince. The folias, like the zambra, was a popular dance. Nowadays in Spain it is generally conceded to be a Portuguese and not a Spanish dance. It would appear to have been more Moorish than anything else, but further investigation will have to be made to determine where and when it originated. At present relatively little is known about its roots.

Open-air dance displays were highly favoured and were sometimes of a competitive nature. They drew distinguished audiences and the following description gives some idea of how they were conducted.[12] 'The square in Purchena was suitably decorated in readiness for the dances and carpets had been laid where they were to be performed. Beneath the platform, Abenhumaya was seated in his chair and army officers were seated in a circle around. It was

---

[11]Emilio Garcia Gomez: *Cinco Poetas Musulmanes*, p. 252. (Madrid 1944).
[12]Gines Perez de Hita: *Las guerras civiles de Granada* (1595).

realized that the lute would sound better if played from where he was sitting and so the musician changed places with him. Well-dressed young Moorish boys entered and each danced marvellously. Next appeared another group accompanied by lovely Moorish maidens and Abenhumaya ordered them to dance alone—which they did most elegantly. The last dancer to appear was a native of Purchena whose solo was so brilliantly performed that everybody was held spellbound by her beauty and the elegant "douane" of her dance.'

Beauty, grace and brilliance impressed the writer more than anything and not one word of criticism was forthcoming, which is a pleasant change. Nevertheless we are not told very much about the actual dances; they remain anonymous for in those days many dances were being born, but not all were yet baptized.

While the Moors were thus disporting themselves in the kingdom of Granada and the Moorish south generally, the Christians in Castille and the Christian north ignored them and set about diverting themselves in their own way. The Peninsula was divided into these two parts. There had been a struggle for supremacy going on for some time between Aragon and Castille but as the fourteenth century dawned, Castille emerged as the more powerful kingdom. An exciting time and place to be living in indeed, with both England and France trying to gain control of it. Large bands of mercenary soldiers coming from every corner of Christendom took up residence to help them gain their ends. Both John of Gaunt and the Black Prince were claimants to the Castilian throne and the French were there to prevent any such claim succeeding. Between battles, the foreign expeditionary forces had to be kept amused. Banquets and similar festivities were held in honour of the mercenary leaders, all of whom would be invited to sit with the king of Castille at the royal table. The kingdom was full of strolling players, musicians, tumblers, dancers and actors. There was something for everybody; folk-dancing for the populace and court-dancing for the nobility. These two aspects of regional dancing appeared to be developing simultaneously. The Christian courts became quite as important as centres for the development of the arts generally, as the Moorish courts had been in the past. Professional artists were attached to them; Christian and Moorish singers and dancers together with the technical experts charged with producing, supervising and directing the entertainments. Court functions consisted largely of banquets followed by diversions which included acting, singing and dancing. The courtiers took an active part by performing also. These festivals of aristocratic art occupied the same place in the lives of the nobles as did the popular religious plays in those of the humbler folk. In those days, the nobles lived in their own regions and each one possessed its own court. The fact that so many of these miniature courts existed assured the continuance of this kind of production and there it was that an appreciation for the visual arts was stimulated and, in particular, dancing prospered under these conditions. Only after the advent of the Catholic kings in the fifteenth century did the nobility start to spend large parts of the year at court in the capital, and then this facet of dancing became metropolitan in flavour as the Moorish and Jewish aspects of life faded into the background.

The reign of Ferdinand and Isabella brought established law and order to the land. The Moorish and Jewish aspects of life which had been so prominent in certain parts of Spain in the past receded as the decree went forth that these people must be baptized or leave the country. Many fled, the rest were converted to Catholicism. At that period, it was found that one method of directing the attention of the people to their religion was by means of scenic plays of a sacred nature which contained much mimed movement and dancing. The dancing had to be of a kind that the ordinary folk understood and folk and ritual dances came to be used for proselytizing the illiterate. They made a direct visual appeal and it became quite customary to perform them within the precincts of a church. These dances, strangely enough, were notorious at times, for their 'indecency' and were then hastily suppressed. The ecclesiastical authorities were fastidious about dancing they permitted on cere-monial occasions and kept a sharp eye on the dancers to see that they took no undue liberties with any dance in a religious context. At the first sign of uncontrolled wildness or passion in the dances, which apparently sometimes occurred, the offending measures were at once proscribed. Whilst dancing of a simple, popular kind might be considered very suitable for making the people more aware of their faith, it had to be satisfactorily adapted to religious needs and this took some time.

Throughout the fifteenth and sixteenth centuries this aspect of sacred, popular dancing was practised, and accordingly developed into a dance form of its own, never reaching the point of being included as an actual means of worship as was song. Despite this constant use, dancing always seemed to cause violent criticism; as far as one can judge, mainly on the grounds that it gave too much pleasurable satisfaction to the people who did it! In vain did the champions of the dance cite the ancient custom of dancing in the Temple or the celestial dance of the angels; these outward signs of religious fervour failed to convince the opposition, who roundly condemned it as illicit, immoral and indecent. No satisfactory answer has yet been found to this question and the fact that dancing has survived after so many centuries of attack in this land of dance and dancers, would appear to indicate what a powerful force it is in Spain.

Turning from the past for the moment, one has only to recall that a few years ago, when the 'love duet' from 'El Amor Brujo' was televised in Madrid, it had to be considerably modified before it was accepted as suitable for the televiewers, and this particular dance had been performed with success and without criticism in international theatres for years. Spaniards grumbled, saying that Spain was fifty years behind the times. What they failed to remember was that in this matter, the twentieth-century Watch Committee was merely conforming to Spanish tradition in forbidding anything they considered remotely dubious morally, in terms of dancing, for public exhibition. This official supervision is not confined to Spanish companies only. In 1965, a visiting company appearing at the Zarzuela Theatre, Madrid, was requested to give a dress rehearsal for the powers-that-be, before the opening night's performance, in order that they might be satisfied that costumes, scenery and movements measured up to contemporary Spanish standards of decency.

To return to the sixteenth century and to sum up: life in Spain had assumed a national form with characteristics that could belong to no other country, since they were the outcome of the liberation of the people after years of foreign occupation. Following this trend, the dancing of the country also was being moulded into a Spanish shape. It was segregated; aristocratic dancing was confined to the palaces and homes of the wealthy, while popular dancing, or that belonging to the people, took place just about everywhere—in the taverns, the market places, fairgrounds, and the open tree-shaded squares and outside the churches. When employed for religious purposes, it was modified, losing in the process some of its roughness and noise. As for social dancing, this differed little from that in the rest of Europe; indeed, the roots were closely intertwined and it might be as well now to attempt to classify it. In the next chapter the early days of dance development in Spain will be considered with reference to dance form abroad in the rest of Europe. It will then be seen how it compared with foreign dancing and how this in turn was affected by Spanish influences.

3

Towards the Classification of Spanish Dancing

THE COUNTRIES of Western Europe, in common with the rest of the world, had their own indigenous dances in the Middle Ages. When the Albigensian troubles scattered the troubadours, their dances, the Provençal estampies became popular and later, in the fourteenth century, basse danse[1] was universally performed. Different forms of this appeared both in France and Italy and it is not certain which influenced the other. Naples had been a Spanish possession since 1442 and had become an important centre where Castilian and Aragonese artists and scholars coming to Italy met. Not until one hundred years later did Italian dance influences predominate, and by that time many Spanish elements had been absorbed into Italian dancing. The extent of this influence up to the late sixteenth century has yet to be determined.

A peninsula, no less than an island, encourages narrow, parochial thoughts, and there is a tendency among Spaniards today to imagine themselves existing in a complete state of isolation, inventing dances for which the rest of Europe remains in their debt. Much as one would like to agree with them, this is not so. One of the most fascinating aspects of dance history is the way in which events in many different countries are bound together in social and political history and directly affect dancing. A royal marriage or a military occupation, for example, may be all important.

England and Spain were linked by marriage as far back as 1170

[1]Processional form of dance in which steps were arranged according to rigid rules.

when Eleanor of England, daughter of Henry II, married King Alfonso VIII in Tarrazona. This marriage took place amid scenes of splendour, pomp and ceremony unheard of in Spain in those days since, as one Spanish chronicler remarked: 'The king of England was the most distinguished and magnificent in all Europe'. To celebrate the occasion, the court went to Burgos where great public demonstrations of joy in the form of feasting and much dancing took place. This was not confined to the nobles, but also enjoyed by the large retinues of men-at-arms, servants and courtiers from both countries. These are such stuff as dance history is made on.

At that time, the English were held in high esteem in the Peninsula. Later, early in the fourteenth century, England and Castille were bound by military, political and matrimonial alliances. Indeed, the Duke of Lancaster was pretender to the Castilian throne. Catherine of Lancaster married Henry of Castille and, inversely, both Henry II and Henry III married Provençal princesses. These inter-alliances went on between the two countries until the fifteenth century when Katharine of Aragon became the wife of Henry VIII. This type of interchange was not confined to royal circles. There were long waiting periods in between battles and mercenaries, men-at-arms, archers and pikemen were not slow in availing themselvesof local diversions that were offered in the form of wine, women, song and dance. Thus military alliances too served the useful purpose of making known to people of other lands unfamiliar dances and other ways of performing their own.

In 1432, at the court of Alfonso the Magnanimous in Naples, the Catalans were much admired for their dancing of the cascarda. Most people assume that this is an Italian court dance because the sixteenth-century Italian dancing master, Caroso, thoughtfully recorded quite a number of them for posterity. It is therefore of much interest to find the Spaniards dancing cascardas one hundred and fifty years before the Italians recorded them. Was it the same dance? Of that one cannot be sure at present. Caroso considered it to be a graceful, dignified, aristocratic dance. It began with a sustained reverence, feet together, not turned out, for this position came into existence later. The gentleman removed his hat, bowed

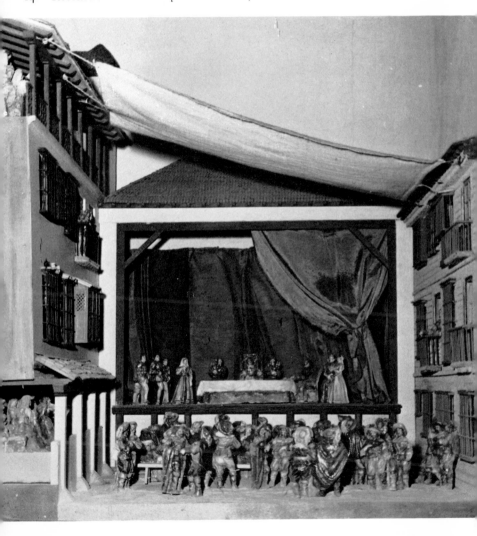

15. Theatrical décor by Rizi, used in the Buen Retiro productions.

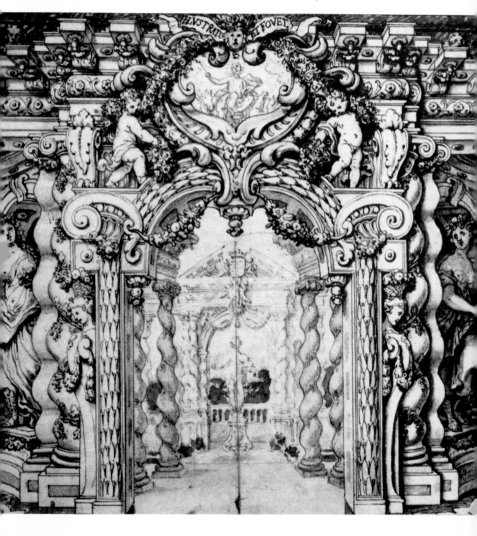

16. Reconstruction of Teatro del Buen Retiro; seventeenth century.

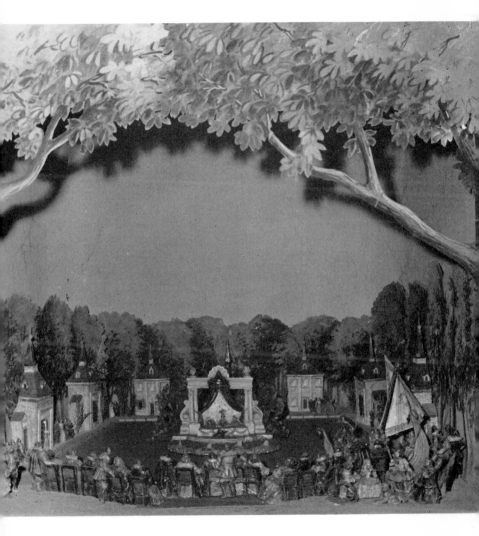

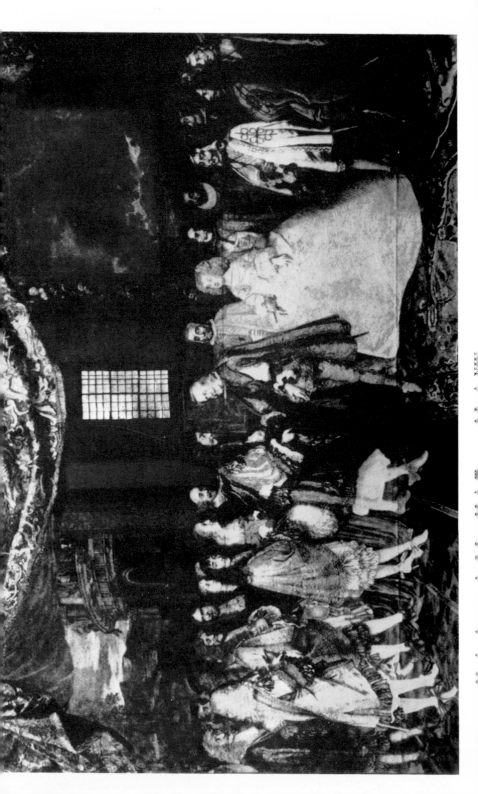

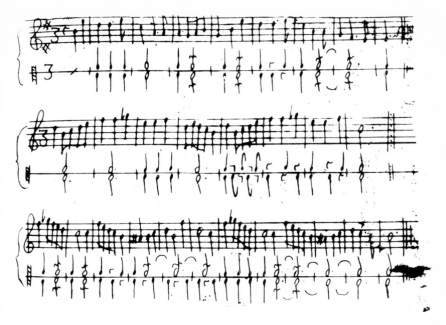

18. Detail from Feuillet's *L'Art de Décrire la Danse*, showing castanet notation.

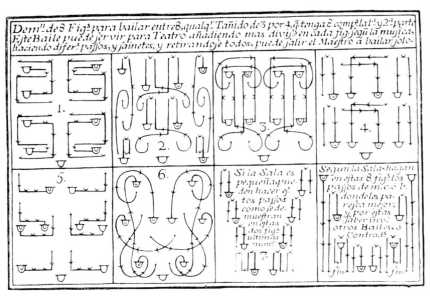

19. Eighteenth century dance notation. Extract from *El Noble Art de Danzar* (1758) showing thirty-six different ground patterns in eight separate figures of dance.

L'ART DE DE'CRIRE

De la batterie des Caſtagnettes.

POur la Batterie des Caſtagnettes, je me ſerviray des Nottes de la Muſique, qui auront les mêmes valeurs & qui ſeront placées aux deux
côtez d'une ſeule ligne, dont les unes ſeront au deſſus & les autres
au deſſous.

Celles qui ſeront au deſſus ſeront pour frapper de la main gauche,
& celles qui ſeront au deſſous ſeront pour frapper de la main droite.

EXEMPLES.

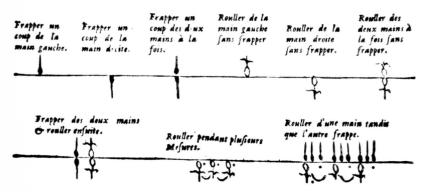

La ligne ſur laquelle les Nottes ſont placées doit être barrée de meſure
en meſure comme dans la Muſique, entre leſquelles barres, ſeront mar-
quées autant de Nottes que l'on doit battre de coups, dans chaque meſures auſquelles on donnera les valeurs convenables aux meſures de l'Air.

Il doit auſſi avoir au commencement de cette ligne une eſpece de
Clef, qui ne ſervira ſeulement que pour en marquer le commencement, afin de pouvoir marquer enſuite le ſigne de meſure de l'air, &
les temps qu'il faudra compter, en cas qu'il y en ait.

EXEMPLE.

20. Explanation of castanet notation showing how it is to be used in
conjunction with music. *Extract from L'Art de Décrire.*

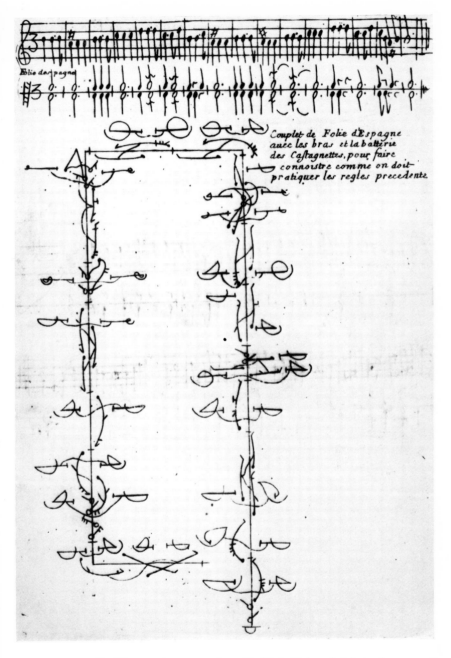

Couplet de Folie d'Espagne
auec les bras et la batterie
des Castagnettes, pour faire
connoistre comme on doit
pratiquer les regles precedente.

21. 'Folie d'Espagne'—extract from *Feuillet's L'Art : de Décrire la Danse* showing ground pattern of dance and castanet notation.

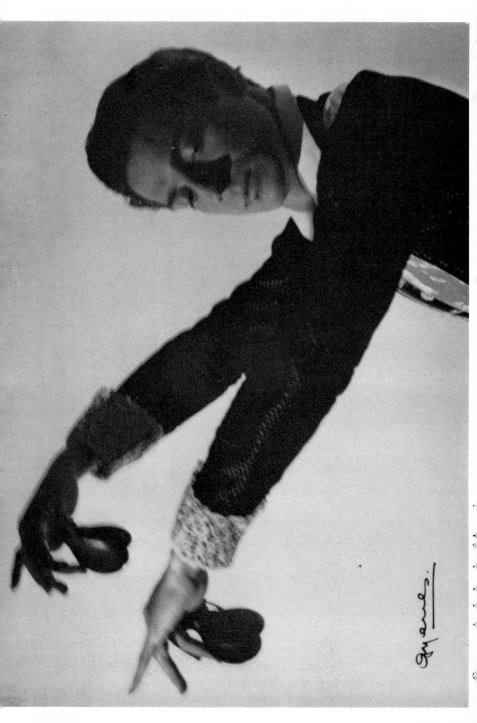

and replaced it before dancing. In the first figure, the dancers, side by side, moved round each other with the same simple walking steps and ended where they began—side by side. The second figure was the same, only the dancers finished differently—facing each other. A refrain with elaborate honours followed. In the third figure, the man danced alone and in the fourth, the girl performed her solo. Then the couple danced the refrain together. The dance continued with the dancers performing sixteen bars together and finally ended with the eighteen-bar refrain as in the other figures. Italian cascardas were danced by two men and a girl or simply by one man and his girl partner. The titles of Caroso's cascardas nearly all pertained to love, Cupid, or both.

Much patient and original research has been done in England in an attempt to discover in what way the Spanish and Italian cascardas resembled each other. In Spain, there appears to be no information available at present. The distinguished Catalan folklorist, the late Joan Amades, had never heard of the dance, but thought that it might have been connected with the cascabeles—a dance of Pyrrhic origin, performed by men only. The victorious entry of the Catalans into Naples suggested this. It does not sound from this that it was related to the Italian conception of the dance. Don Joan discounted any possibility of the Catalan version being a linked dance, for the Church at that time was doing its best to stamp out anything that brought the sexes together in a dance or could be construed to be of an amorous nature in any way. This is an interesting point inviting further research for it appears to be a dance of Spanish origin and, if so, the antecedents of a good many other dances recorded by Italians will have to be re-examined, their origin reappraised, and the results could change the whole face of modern dance history.

Intermarriage between the royal houses of Europe, already pointed out, meant much coming and going between the countries concerned, with many visitors of different nationalities, all of whom had to be amused. Since there is no language barrier in dancing, what better way could there be than this? Many brought their own dances or variations with them, along with other native customs. Some of the dances took root, others did not, only enjoying perhaps a temporary vogue, then disappearing without leaving a trace. The kings of Spain were lovers of art and it was quite customary for them to send emissaries abroad in search of information, or to invite foreign experts to come to Spain to instruct and entertain the Spanish Court. Juan I of Aragon, a great music lover, sent word to the Duke of Burgundy that he would like the famous Johan de Orgurns to come immediately, bringing with him the book in which the estampies[2] were recorded.

In 1380, Juan I married a French princess, Violant de Bar. This youthful queen was overpowered by the austerity, sobriety and strict etiquette which she found at the Aragonese court, and wrote home to say so. When she was expecting her first baby, she particularly yearned for the gaiety of the French Court and asked her mother to tell her what they were dancing in France just then. She longed to see some of the latest dances and begged her mother to send some French courtiers to cheer her up by showing them to her. Her mother replied that there was a very lively little dance in vogue at home called the 'pampalona'. It was somewhat strenuous and therefore not to be recommended to Her Royal Highness in her present condition—she would be well advised to restrict herself to the more sedate measures of the Aragonese court for the present. But of course somebody would come and show her the dance (pl. 5).

The only specimen of a pampalona[3] I came across in Spain was that in a collection of basses danses in the National Library, Madrid. The author of this document was a young lawyer named Antonio Arena, a student at Avignon University in 1510. He claimed that these dances were most uncommon and performed chiefly at banquets and similar festivities. He suggested to dancers that if, by any chance, they should lose their place in the dance, to keep moving at all costs, for there was nothing worse than standing still and looking foolish.

Belonging to the late fifteenth century, the first Spanish document to give some valuable clues concerning the nature of fifteenth-

[2]Judging from the Harley Ms. 978 (c. 1240; British Museum) estampies were hardly distinguishable from the common branles. The one variation by which the estampie music may be recognized occurs in the 'branle simple' where every fourth unit contains five bars instead of six.

[3]R. c. ss. d. r. c. ss. d. ss. r. c. ss. ddd. r. c. ss. d. ss. r. c.

century dances is the Cervera manuscript which may be found at Lerida, Aragon. Most of the dances here recorded are clearly in the French tradition. This record is a great help towards understanding the steps because they were accurately described and adhered to the French rules; singles must be in pairs, doubles and reprises must be uneven—one, three or five. Every measure must begin and end with a reverence and a branle. The Spanish dances were peculiar in suggesting back as well as forward movements on the singles and reprises. Of special interest to English readers is the presence of 'Anglaterra' with 'Castille' and 'Bassa Morisca'. Also of particular interest is the document in the library of Salisbury Cathedral, very similar to that from Cervera. For the purpose of comparison, a description of 'Filles a Marier' in both manuscripts is given at the end of the book (Appendix B, p. 190), from which it will be seen that they are almost identical (pls. 7, 8).

It should not be assumed from this, that all Spanish dancing was predominantly French in the fifteenth century. Although the crowns of Leon and Castille had been unified by the marriage of Ferdinand and Isabella, after the Moors had been driven out of Spain, oriental traditions lingered on in most things, including Spanish dancing. Indeed, they have never been completely abandoned. It was in the Christian north that European influences prevailed over those from the East but the indigenous dancing of the people remained the solid foundation of Spanish dance in the Peninsula. Diverse external influences were repeatedly superimposed upon that solid base but never obliterated the national dances. It may well have been this constant state of flux that prevented Spanish dancing from becoming static and devitalized. This became clear in the sixteenth century as different types of Spanish dances began to emerge. Before proceeding to classify them, let us turn for a moment to the construction of early dance form, since all the diverse types of social dances everywhere were the offshoots of this.

The first dance about which we can be precise was the carole, a linked dance accompanied by song; there might be a tambour or some thrumming instrument to mark the time, but the song comprised the music. There were two forms of carole, the file or farandole, and the round dance, the branle. The farandole was introduced by the Greeks who had settlements in Catalonia and Marseilles. Traces of these dances may still be found in these districts, which were formerly part of medieval Provence and stretched far beyond the bounds of modern Provence. It was danced by all classes, although it may be supposed that there was some difference if the accompanying song was a folk-song. As the steps were only running or walking ones, almost any music was suitable, for there was no need for precise rhythms as in branles. This is why it is difficult to identify old farandole music. Although there were no known steps, there were figures, the most important being 'threading the needle' which involves the dancers passing under each other's arms, and whenever this figure is found, we may suspect a farandole in the background.

The other form of carole was the branle[4]—a round dance, which always included singing, and in which the dancers were linked. There were other round dances, especially in England, but not belonging to this class. Where the farandole weaved round at the pleasure of the leader, the branle, or round dance, was a closed circle turning to the left or to the right for the sake of variety. It was more limited in movement, but it developed rhythmic patterns. It also contained a swaying movement which accounts for the name 'branle'. Branles were arranged in suites of increasing pace. There were were *branles simples*, *doubles* and *gais*.

As the farandole[5] was the national dance of Provence, so the branle was characteristic of France. The prevalence of branle rhythms in troubadour music suggests that it must also have been danced in Provence which, in the twelfth century, was not part of France, but linked with Aragon and Catalonia.

The medieval mind was devoted to systems and all dances had to be reduced to a set of rules that were easy to follow. Generally speaking, the dances were in triple time and consisted of figures rather than steps; such steps as did exist were mostly of a walking variety, performed at different speeds and designed to take up an

---

[4]A 'branle' consists of a dance unit and its accompanying music unit, which are repeated over and over again as long as the dance lasts.

[5]Generally speaking we owe the development of steps to the branles whilst figures derive from the farandole.

even amount of music. Their pattern could be that of a winding line, as in processional dances, a circle, as in round dances; or it might consist of dancers linking hands, as in a chain dance. Round, chain and processional dances were the three basic types of dance current in the Middle Ages and were danced everywhere; in the homes of the nobility on ceremonial occasions and also in the open air by the people, at their rustic gatherings. Although fundamentally alike in construction, the popular form of the dances was coarser and danced in a rougher manner, heavier in quality because of the weight of the footwear. Remains of the dances used in medieval morality plays which were simple in design may be seen in the ground patterns of theatrical choreography still in use today.

The first development in dancing was the breaking up of linked dances into small units of two or three dancers. This change seems to have taken place in Provence, as a refinement of troubadour influence. The dances which resulted were the estampies. They preserved the divisions of the branle suites and added simple patterns, with slight variations in steps. There were estampies *simples*, *doubles* and *gais*. These developments appeared clearly in France, but were not quite so apparent in other countries. As far as Spain was concerned, little has remained to guide us. That Juan I of Aragon particularly asked to see the books in which the estampies were noted, suggests that in fourteenth-century Aragon, the estampies were something of a novelty. Spanish authorities on the subject in the last century did not consider that estampies had ever taken root in Spain, and there is still no evidence to show that they persisted there, either in folk- or court-dancing. The distinguished Spanish musical historian Don Felipe Pedrell sought in vain for details of estampies, both in court literature and collections of ancient lute music. In his opinion an estampie was simply a dance in which the accent was strongly marked by beating the feet on the ground. The name was derived from this action— *estampar* meaning in Spanish 'to stamp the feet'.

This may come as a shock to those English dance researchers accustomed to believe that estampies formed the basis upon which European dance form was constructed, and they may well wonder what took its place in the early development of Spanish dance form.

As the rule of coming forward on the left foot and back on the right was strict and unalterable in estampies, so it was in basse danse. In basse danse,[6] the entire dance really consisted of movements of courtesy. Taking into account the heavy costumes worn by the ladies in the fourteenth and fifteenth centuries it is obvious why basse danse could not be anything other than very formal.

In the fourteenth century, basse danse or 'baja' in Spanish became very fashionable but, like other dances already referred to, different countries evolved their own variations of the dance. The Italian version of basse danse was entirely different from the French. The rules were different and it was not influenced by the branles. It was closer to the farandole and arranged to be danced in small rooms; unlike the French, which was designed to be performed in the spacious rooms of the French *châteaux* or royal palaces. The Spanish version appears to have been influenced by France rather than Italy. An even, four-bar phrase was typical.

Here again we are presented with divergent opinions on what Spanish basse danse really was. In Spanish, *baja* means low and the consensus of Spanish opinion is that this name indicates that the dance emanated from Low Germany, or Flanders. By the same reasoning the *alta* is presumed to have been brought to Spain from High Germany, by foreigners. The title 'Spanish alta' is really most confusing and quite misleading for there may have been nothing Spanish about it! 'Spanish' might have been a means of distinguishing certain variations of a dance then universally performed. It might even have been appended by the Italians to distinguish the variations they saw the Spaniards doing in Italy, that were distinct from their own and, when recording the alta, they merely applied the term 'Spanish alta' to distinguish it from their own preconceived notions of the dance. It is also quite possible that it may have been a dance specially commissioned by a Spaniard. One thing is certain, a long and unfruitful search covering the whole of Spain, revealed no Spanish document concerning a 'Spanish alta'.

That great authority on early Spanish dances, Don Garcia

---

[6]Basically, the steps were grouped by arbitrary rules into 'measures'. Every measure began with: 2 singles (ss) forward continued with 3 or 5 doubles (ddd or ddddd) and ended with 1 or 3 reprises (r or rrr) and a branle (b).

Matos, was consulted and the only example he knew of in Spain, was an early alta in a collection of fifteenth and sixteenth century Spanish music entitled *Cancionero de Barbiere*. This consisted of thirty-eight bars of music in triple time composed for three instruments. No steps of the dance were given. An 'alta' is described in a manuscript at the Academia Réal de Historia, Madrid, but the authorities there informed me that it was probably of Italian origin. The fifteenth-century Italian dancing master, Domenico de Ferrarra,[7] recorded a 'Spanish Alta' which he likened to a pas de brabant. This tallies with the Spanish conviction that it came from abroad and was an intermediate form of a tordion. It has been claimed that the Pas de Brabant became the galliard and possibly this Spanish alta may have had the same rhythm and thus became the pavane, as later, pavane music was written in galliard time. Outside Spain this is a controversial subject, but in Spain itself the alta is considered to be a dance of non-Spanish origin.

Italian masters have to be referred to for information regarding Spanish dances because they, unlike the Spaniards in those early days, recorded what they taught. This does not mean that their teaching was necessarily confined to Italian dances only. Dance instruction was much the same everywhere in Europe in Domenico's time. Broadly speaking, it consisted of not permitting the knees to sag and keeping the thigh muscles well braced. These very stiff knees gave to the movements an appearance of stiffness and were very characteristic of early court dancing. The Spaniards had been in occupation of a large part of Italian territory and it is probable that some of the dance material collected by the Italian masters may have been Spanish; yet another matter awaiting closer investigation.

The teaching of dancing had been regarded as a serious profession throughout the Middle Ages in Spain. The Spanish dancing masters had their own guild which was a professional brotherhood, similar to guilds belonging to the other arts and crafts. In order to become a member of their guild and qualify as a dancing master, aspirants had to pass a test, to prove that they had an adequate

[7]Domenico de Ferrarra was composing figure dances c. 1440, designed to be danced indoors.

knowledge of their subject and also the ability to teach it. It may be concluded from this that some method of teaching existed, but as references are somewhat vague, we do not yet know what it was. The fifteenth-century Spanish dances adhered to a set form as they did in the rest of Europe. They were not spontaneous outbursts or improvised, therefore anyone wishing to be proficient would have to take the trouble to learn and practise them; in other words, methodical dance instruction at that time was indispensable.

Dancing was transformed after it was brought indoors on to well-laid floors of wood or marble pavements; then, technique commenced; simply at first, as the dancers, rising on to the toes, lightened the quality of the movement. The old steps remained for a long time, but showed a tendency to be split up, making for quicker footwork. Even in the days of the early branles, there had been dances of mixed rhythms which took sections from different branles and combined them. This was also done with estampies. Dance steps had been based on singles and doubles, which stepped on the first beat of the bar up to the sixteenth century. After this, a change took place, when music was divided into short bars which meant that the steps were quicker, taking only one bar instead of four. Sixteenth-century France was still dancing branles with the addition of mime. Basse danse had gone out in the first quarter of the century, leaving the pavane, galliard, the volta and alleman, a German legacy from the fourteenth century. In Italy, a more elaborate system appears to have prevailed, as Domenico based his theories on separate musical forms: basse danse, salterello, quaternaria and piva. They had their own musical values and steps, but when they were all combined into one dance, a new form was born called 'ballo' or 'balletto'. This form could have any number of dancers of either sex; the steps in themselves were not difficult but the manner of performing them called for the utmost subtlety. It is not yet known exactly when, nor where, these changes of rhythm and technique first took place; there was a general leaning towards this sort of innovation throughout the fifteenth century and the French and Italian dancing masters thoughtfully recorded them.

Domenico's style was elaborated in Italy, but, as has been observed, Italy was partially occupied by Spain then and so it was natural to find strong Spanish influences there. The form of the dance that evolved was one in which the partners took turns in dancing the variations, of varying difficulty, between short linking passages which they danced together. The ballo or balletto continued with their mixed rhythms and basse danse remained longer in Italy than elsewhere. In France and England, the galliard acquired a prominent position, until it became so acrobatic that a change was necessary. This came from France, although there is some evidence to suggest that there was Spanish influence here too. The new style was devoid of leaps, depended on instep control and was very sustained. The French and the English, like the Italians, avoided knee-bending and the toes turned out in the sideways movement in the new type of branle. Known as courantes and canaries, the new dances were sustained and Spanish in style, with dragging and beaten steps. Little was said about the gavotte but there can be no doubt that the sarabande was danced socially.

Oh! the mysterious sarabande! So much has been written about it in so many different terms that one can but wonder how many forms of the dance there were. If the court sarabande resembled the dance of the same name, danced in Spain, it is most extraordinary that it had to go outside the Peninsula to be accepted socially. Anybody in Spain caught dancing the sarabande would be flogged, for it was forbidden by law. In 1583, a decree went forth to the effect that, in addition to being flogged, the men would be condemned to the galleys and the women banished from the land! The Spaniards, with nonchalant indifference to the law, cheerfully went on dancing the sarabande until well on in the seventeenth century. Moralists and theologians continued to thunder against it, but their threats appear to have fallen on deaf ears. One of the leading antagonists was Padre Mariano who claimed that the sarabande had done more harm than the plague; he explained why! It was a very exciting dance in which the arms and castanets were never still. How very interesting to find at that early date, the upper part of the body coming in for criticism; hitherto, the undulating movements of the hips had caused most of the murmurings against the dance. In the sixteenth century, the bodices of dresses were very *décolleté* and it has been suggested that the movement of the women's breasts perturbed the critics, which seems as good an explanation as any other. The Spanish version of the dance obviously had little in common with the social sarabande known abroad as a slow and stately measure. The foreign form may have been some sort of galliard but, as yet, there is no proof of this or any examples before the French dancing master, Pécour's, time.[8]

We come now to the social dances of Spain, which may be roughly divided into three categories; those belonging to the Church, the Palace and the People. No less than in foreign dances, they adhered to a set form, upon which national elements were superimposed. Any classification of Spanish dance would be incomplete if it underestimated the prominent part religion plays in the lives of the Spanish people who, since they danced as well as sang in praise of God, made this aspect of Spanish dancing important.

Spain has been called the 'Land of Faith'—with good reason for faith was everywhere present as it continues to be today. Throughout the ages, dancing in Spain has been closely connected with the Faith; to such an extent that at one point dancing in church had to be proscribed, was then condemned in religious processions and in the fifteenth century it was finally forbidden. There was a perfectly sound reason for these extreme measures; the dances had become altogether too wild so clerics decided that dancing of this uncontrolled kind was not a fitting or proper manner in which to worship. Only in the sixteenth century did ritual dances begin to reappear in the 'Autos da Fé' and since then have been in continuous use in religious processions and ceremonies (pl. 6).

One of the most interesting forms of sacred dancing was that found in the 'bailes de cofradía', so called because they were performed when transporting holy relics from one shrine to another. These dances belonged to the processional group and were invariably of a slow, solemn nature. This quality by no means applied to all sacred dances, however, for in some of the religious plays, for example, other types of dance were included and even the grotesque element was not despised. This was very evident in the mojigangas which are of extreme interest to dancers today, for they were

[8]Pécour et Feuillet: Recueil de Danses: Paris, 1709.

distinctly theatrical in conception. Disguised as animals or giants, the dancers performed dances consisting entirely of figures and containing no steps. Very frequently a mojiganga was pure burlesque. Mojigangas formed part of the Easter, Christmas and Corpus Christi processions and were also used as a finale to the type of play then known as an 'Auto Sacramentale'. There was a lot of dancing of various kinds in these 'Autos'; zapateadores, sword dancers, and the cascabel dancers, whose leaders carried a small flag—for this was formerly the dance of victory, performed after wars. Fandangos were also much prized and a *pas de deux* performed by the dancers representing the Holy Ghost and the Virgin Mary in one of these plays was no other than a fandango *à deux*. It was quite permissible and indeed usual to add mimed movement and gesture to the dances. In the fifteenth and sixteenth centuries, a large proportion of the people was illiterate and this combination of music, song, dance and gesture, was a visual aid serving to convey the message of faith to the masses. These performances were, in fact, ballets in embryo. The themes were based on simple, allegorical stories of a religious nature; the dances were those belonging to the round, chain, processional groups, or of a collective variety. There were also solos, duets, trios, and quartets for the leading characters. Pantomime was freely used and the grotesque element was rarely absent. Since the whole object was to instruct while entertaining the crowd, these little ballets had to make a direct appeal, comprehensible to all the spectators. Settings had to be familiar to countrymen as well as town dwellers. One such piece was set in booths in a fairground. Figures representing the Virgin Mary occupied one booth, Jesus Christ another, and the rest were taken over by the Seven Deadly Sins. The crowd naturally veered towards the latter in preference to the Holy Family, who, after expressing their fury at lack of business in a *pas de deux*, drove out their competitors with whips, no less!

The same leading characters recurred in this type of spectacle, the Holy Family, the Deadly Sins, Adam, the Good Shepherd, and the Archangels. The *corps de ballet* consisted of saints, sinners, nymphs, shepherds, the heavenly bodies, and there were also symbolic figures representing such things as vice and virtue, peace and war, cupid and flowers and so forth. The design of the dances was unpretentious: farandoles, weaving in and out in a maze, or groups of three or four on each side of the stage crossing and recrossing in various directions. They were sometimes accompanied by singing, or sometimes the dancers first sang, then danced to the same tune. There were also 'las danzas habladas', a combination of dance and speech which was very frequently seen in the sixteenth century.

As in the past, similar religious functions are still to be seen in Spain today. Open-air pageants, religious processions and plays do take place, but in a modified form and it is doubtful whether the artists taking part in them receive the same solicitous care as did their forebears. That they were well fed on the day of performance is made very clear in a memorandum coming from the archives of Toledo Cathedral dated 1454. They were to be given a light luncheon before the actual performance and a more substantial meal after the event. On the day of Our Lady, lunch or snack consisted of: 'cakes, grapes, figs, bread and wine'; dinner was quite a luxurious affair: 'beef, geese, melons, grapes, and rice with cinnamon and spice.' Prices were appended, and other important items mentioned were: 'Cabbage, carrots, fish, eggs, bread, wine, wood and coal for heating'. Instructions were given regarding the type of dances required, what costumes were to be worn and the appropriate musical accompaniment—tambourine, bagpipes, etc. One senses an air of professionalism already, in these religious manifestations.

We pass now to a type of Spanish dancing of quite a different nature. This belongs to the second category mentioned earlier. These dances were of an aristocratic nature and appropriately called 'bailes palaciegos', doubtless an allusion to the place where they were performed, which was generally indoors in the homes of the nobility. They were not always grave and dignified. On occasions they could be very bright and lively. They were usually set dances of the pavane, galliard type which everyone was expected to know. Not only were they danced for pleasure by the guests at parties, they were extensively used in the masques held at court, and in the entertainments then becoming fashionable at banquets and similar festivities. They were accompanied by lute, harp or song and the

Spaniards were very fond of using verse as an accompaniment. At the masque given in 1559 in honour of the marriage of Philip II and Isabel de Valois, the verses were composed by no less a person than Ronsard.

In the Renaissance period it was fun to fit in as much movement as possible into a musical phrase; a contrast with medieval days, when an even bar of music took an even phrase of movement. This led to some of the dances becoming veritable feats of virtuosity, which were reserved for the gentlemen while the ladies looked on admiringly. The galliard was the dance in which they shone. At a ball held in 1560 at Guadalajara, Don Diego de Cordova was reported to have danced a galliard that 'lasted some time'. This can be well believed when it was remembered that Don Diego was probably showing off his technical prowess in some difficult variations that had been specially arranged for him. He had doubtless put in many hours of practice perfecting the acrobatic feats then called for: somersaults and chest rolls, high jumping steps and brilliant twirls and whirls in the air. It is worth noting in passing that English courtiers then earned for us the title of the 'Dancing English' because they were reputed to 'jump higher and turn more than dancers from other lands'.

Sometimes the pavane and galliard might be joined together to form a contrast. The older members of the company might dance the dignified processional pavane, then discreetly withdraw while the young people let themselves go on the galliard. The Spanish pavane was a great favourite; the French knew it, so did the English, and Queen Elizabeth liked it so well that she commanded English composers to write pavanes specially for her. Many foreign versions of the dance were in existence for it was danced with great enthusiasm in aristocratic homes all over Europe. There is an example of an Italian pavane—a manuscript of the early sixteenth century[9]—in the Academia Réal de Historia, Madrid, useful for the purpose of comparison with the Spanish version.

It was clear that the Spaniards wielded considerable influence over court-dancing in sixteenth-century England, where good dancing was admired by all who moved in court circles. These

[9] Ms. in folio. r 25. Folio 4290.

dances were based on estampies, basse danse and branles and were
therefore very similar everywhere. Spain maintained close contact
with Italy and Provence throughout the fifteenth century and the
dances reflect influences from these countries. It was in the sixteenth
century that a more highly individualized, national style of dancing
began to emerge, when more homespun elements taken from
popular dances began to creep into the sedate refinement of aristocratic dancing. Then one became aware of the diversity in the
Spanish variations of the European court dances; they set a style
followed at the Spanish court and, later, adopted by others in
Europe.

If one is in search of diversity in the realm of dancing, no better
source may be found than in that of the Spanish people. The
popular dances of Spain still vary from region to region, but much
folk material has been lost with the passage of time. In the sixteenth
century, the ordinary people were far removed from the aristocrats
and so was their style of dancing. This was governed to a large
extent by the kind of clothing and the shoes they wore. All peasants
did not go about all of the time in bare feet as some people seem to
think. One visitor was aware that to dance court dances in hobnailed
boots would be incongruous, to say the least! That sixteenth-century
visitor was a court official sent to the Asturias, in the north of Spain,
on official business and this is what he observed: 'The women were
badly made; hunched shoulders, short necks, big heads, puckered
brows and eyes like slits. Dilated nostrils and big mouths, copious
bosoms and abundant rumps, spacious waists, coarse hair and
hands splayed like those of a duck. They wore narrow skirts, mid-
calf in length, revealing their backsides, and high-fastening
hob-nailed boots, made from roughly tanned cowhide, not smooth
cordova leather. How I wished that I could have seen those ladies
dancing a pavanilla italiana, a galliard, alleman, or a saltarello. Alas,
only a cornet was available in those parts and so my wish was never
granted.'

The last category of Spanish dances to be considered is that
known as folk-dancing. These dances were usually associated with
the open air and therefore bore the name of 'bailes de plaza'. It is
not difficult to conjure up a picture of a French, English or Italian

nobleman of the Renaissance dancing, but when it comes to visual-izing the Spanish populace, it is quite another matter. Naturally, the peasants in their bright costumes spring to mind at once, but what about the labourers, artisans and craftsmen? The Christians and Moriscos—those Moors who had remained in Spain and been converted to Christianity—to say nothing of that heterogeneous population consisting of foreign workers, French and Italians, mingled with Turkish and Berber prisoners-of-war brought back to work in Spain as slaves? Then there were the rogues, vagabonds, beggars and gypsies with no specified home or occupation—a very mixed, colourful lot of people—all with their own way of dancing. The last group even had their own dances, impressing the writers of the time by their impropriety; these were called 'bailes picarescos'.

In sixteenth-century Spain, a tremendous resurgence of interest in folk-dancing swept through the country like a tornado and influenced every other type of dancing then in existence there. Folk influences penetrated the entire field of Spanish dancing whether religious, ritualistic, theatrical, or social, i.e. belonging to the ballroom. One has not to look far for a reason. The Spanish people were savouring the experience of being one nation, with one crown and one religion. National customs began to take precedence over all others. The Moors had been driven out, the reign of the Catholic kings established, and the population converted to one faith. Gone was the tyranny of the feudal lords and the old bailes de feodalism gave way to a new uninhibited kind of movement. The Spanish folk literally danced for joy. A relic of those times exists in an old dance still in existence in Catalonia, where one group of dancers represent the rich, another the poor; they dance together and then change places with each other. This was the sort of device used as a means of expressing in movement, in dance form, the pride the Spaniards now felt in their new-found union. The fore-runner of what is today called *pas de deux* was introduced, with the male partners lifting their girls high into the air—considered very advanced in those days. In Spain this was interpreted to mean that the dignity of the woman was now elevated, since men no longer had supreme rights over her.

Popular dances were fraught with a new significance and, no

longer hampered by cumbersome costumes as in the past, the Spaniards threw formality to the winds, and disported themselves on every possible occasion, expressing delight in their new-found liberty in their dances. The most important happening in the development of Spanish dancing in the sixteenth century was the tremendous impact it seemed to make upon the lives of the Spanish people of all classes. The happy release from centuries of occupation by foreigners and the added turmoil of civil wars, burst forth in a spirit of jubilation that found an outlet in art and music, song, poetry and dancing. Dancing in particular was revitalized and transformed into a savagely robust, ebullient, national stream of energy. New force was infused into the stereotyped dances of high society, with their hitherto discreet harp, lute, or mandoline accompaniment. Those dances became completely overshadowed by boisterous folk-dances with their banging tambourines, rattling castanets, snapping fingers and stamping feet. These noisy accompaniments slowly made their way into more formal surroundings and court-dancing became less reserved and infinitely brighter as a result. Among the more noisy types of Spanish dancing was that called the 'zapateo'. In the sixteenth century, this popular form of dancing far exceeded any other in favour and zapateadores were in great demand for sacred representations. Zapateadores were in a class apart from bailadores, and in church records it was quite plainly stated how many dancers were required and, in addition, the number of zapateadores that had to be engaged. Zapateador was the name given to them because they stamped their feet smartly on the ground and in doing so beat out the rhythm. The dance called the 'zapateado' might be elaborated by the zapateador slapping the soles of his feet with the hands, but this had to be done without breaking the rhythm. Today, this type of dance has come down to us in the form of highly stylized zapateados in the theatre and if, in the process of graduating there, they have lost much of their roughness, they have gained in precision. This type of zapateado resembles the steady ticking of a clock, and, unless it is brilliantly done, can be just about as interesting. One thing it has retained, however, is the original quality of noisiness. Cervantes found this sort of dancing very rough and uncouth in his day—understandably when it is remembered that it was then performed on a table in a tavern, a roughly constructed platform, or else in patios and the streets. Zapateadores then would have to stamp considerably harder than present-day stage executants if they wished to be heard above the din made by an average Spanish crowd. That was, after all, part of the excitement of any popular form of entertainment then. Rhythm was the all-important quality and it could not be broken in this form of dancing. Simple sequences of zapateo were refined and added to the social dances of the time and this made them far more interesting to watch and to do, infinitely more intricate to perform and, as they became more involved, they were ultimately incorporated into the developed dance technique of social dance.

Theatrical dancing was still in its infancy. Such theatres as there were, were not good, but zapateadores were much in demand for the performances given in the open air, usually on rugged platforms. Under these difficult conditions, inexpensive, modest little spectacles were presented and they were well within the reach of ordinary citizens. Those early theatres were little more than glorified booths, a continuation of the old ambulatory theatres, rigged up on floats that travelled from town to village, from village to hamlet, bringing modest little acts consisting of zapateadores, acrobats, tumblers, singers, dancers and actors to cheer up the populace (pl. 9). A few simple little props and a whole family of entertainers assured the inhabitants of a complete variety entertainment. They were far removed from the select, private functions held in the homes of the varying degrees of the vast Spanish nobility! There were of course outdoor entertainments on a more ambitious scale; those for example, designed to honour distinguished visitors, or to divert the court during a royal progress. Philip II attended one of this kind and this was the impression made upon the spectator:

At each end of the palace, a platform had been erected, for the musicians who were to accompany the dances with drums, fifes, and similar low instruments. The company, having eaten, the mechanical trades showed them their dances. In order to have a good view, the ladies were seated near the door of the palace. Each trade had a dance of its own and one tried to outdo the other by presenting something unusual. One group consisted of well-grown little nigger boys who, climbing on to each others' shoulders, stuck out their tongues or threw figs at the spectators to make them laugh. A group of labourers presented a very good dance and another showed some dancing giants who danced to such good effect that a twenty-five-foot wall on the river bank adjoining the palace collapsed and some of the dancers were plunged into the river. With such games the day ended.[10]

Nothing, so far, has been said about the gypsies. Yet they were very much in evidence in the sixteenth century. Cervantes refers to them dancing in *La Gitanilla*. He mentioned four gypsy boys and men making an entrance. They were led by a 'great' gypsy dancer. Above the din of the drums and castanets, a murmur of approval could be heard as a pretty gypsy girl appeared. Drums, castanets and gypsies sound like a baile picaresco. Nothing specific is said about the dance the gypsies performed, but sixteenth-century writings make it obvious that the gypsies then were already known in Spain for their dancing. What is not so clear, is what exactly they were dancing. They may have brought their own dances with them, but it is equally probable that they copied the popular Spanish dances they discovered in whichever region they happened to find themselves. The gypsies and their dances will be discussed at greater length later in the book. For the present, it is sufficient to observe that they were already well installed in the Peninsula and, like everyone else who wished to settle in Spain at that time, they were obliged to become Roman Catholics. Church records reveal that gypsies were paid to dance in religious plays when required and, that being the case, they doubtless had to dance whatever was needed, arranged for them by whoever was in charge of the production. It is more than likely that, when accepting Spanish religious beliefs, they found it expedient to adopt Spanish dances as well as the Spanish manner of dancing. This is another interesting point of research awaiting investigation.

After the arrival of the Catholic kings, and the conversion of all the inhabitants of Spain to Catholicism, the survival of medieval mystery plays was guaranteed at a time when their death knell had

[10]Enrique Cock, in *Relación de Felipe II*.

sounded elsewhere in Europe. The official sponsoring of this type of representation proved to be an excellent thing for certain facets of Spanish dancing. Had they not been conserved in this way, they might have been lost for ever. The continuous practice thus afforded to the dancers of working together in these highly-organized religious performances meant that a standard of dancing was set and maintained. Furthermore, the fact that it was encouraged and officially controlled, suggests that it was useful as an educative force. The Church, supervising and thus sheltering this particular aspect of Spanish dancing, did not hesitate to forbid any that they considered to be too sensual. There was no chance of the dances used in a religious way being anything other than decorous; therefore the only form that was liable to get out of hand, or become wildly abandoned, was that of a social nature, whether danced by the 'folk' or the nobility, and this is what became the butt of constant ecclesiastical attack.

To sum up: up to the fourteenth century Spanish dancing developed slowly, but between then and the sixteenth, a period of rapid change set in. The linked dances had been broken into sections: estampies, branles and basses danses had all become something else. Once the dances were brought indoors on to suitable floors, a technique began to be evolved from the early steps, rising on the toes as in dances like the pavane, jumps, leaps and turns, as in the galliard, lifting the girls into the air as in the españoleta. All these developments heralded the birth of Spanish dance technique. With the arrival of the sixteenth century, duple time was added to triple and, with this useful rhythmical adjunct, there could be more invention in the rhythmic pattern of the steps, a great innovation at the time, that contributed much to the progress of dancing. Clothing was lighter than formerly and so the dancers could move with corresponding freedom. These two factors also helped to enlarge the scope of the dances. The appearance of more and better theatres giving regular performances mainly of a popular nature to a considerably larger public than hitherto was an advantage that vastly improved the quality of stage dancing. As many more functions of a theatrical nature were given, dance production had to be increasingly original and the dances more diverse. The outcome of this accelerated dance activity was that choreographic design became infinitely more varied.

By far the most striking feature of Spanish dancing in the sixteenth century was the extraordinarily powerful influence the popular Spanish dances exerted upon all other forms, primarily as a result of being constantly employed in religious plays, pageants and processions. As the people had more time and opportunity to enjoy dancing and saw more of it in public than formerly, their taste for it grew. This seemed to be a natural reaction after Spain had been reconverted to Christianity; indeed it may well have been a deliberate attempt to eliminate, as far as possible, Moorish customs from their daily life and so make the Spaniards more aware of their own. Dancing, like bull-fighting, became a national occupation at that period and nobody could avoid being made to realize it.

The most curious phenomenon of all was the way in which folk-dancing imposed itself, ultimately to sweep away social barriers, thus encroaching upon every other type of Spanish dancing. Always controlled however, whenever ritual dancing was involved, this dancing was never permitted to become too unruly. The ever vigilant Church saw to it that sacred dances conformed to their requirements and, by keeping them within a religious framework, never allowed them to deviate from set standards. In this, they rendered great service to dance form. One has only to read the criticisms levelled at the time to realize the direction in which popular dancing was veering in the hands of the 'folk'.

Social dancing in Spain had followed European trends for a long time before Spanish folk elements were amalgamated with them. Dancing at court did not suddenly develop a 'Spanish style'. It took some time to evolve and the result was the gradual merging of popular folk elements with the dance material already existing in court dances. It was a most significant change when a renovated form of Spanish dance finally replaced that coming from France, Italy and elsewhere, at court.

The underlying differences resided in the variation of character-istic Spanish rhythms; native steps—notably a refined version of zapateo which were beaten steps—and a distinctive manner of performing them. There was a vaguely oriental feeling in the quality of the movements and the use of the castanets for accompanying the dances conclusively hispanicized them. At the end of the sixteenth century the rest of Europe became aware of these dance influences and by the time the seventeenth century dawned, Spanish dance forms were coming into fashion among European dancing masters and in the aristocratic dances of the day.

This important happening came at an opportune moment, for everywhere in Europe dancing was developing at a great pace and Spanish roots became closely intertwined with those belonging to other countries. That a developed type of national dancing, a type that could belong to no other country, should emerge in sixteenth-century Spain was to be expected, in view of the peculiar social conditions then prevailing. The unification of the Spanish people is sufficient explanation in itself, after so many centuries of upheaval and foreign occupation in parts of Spain. The dance was a positive force in helping to weld the nation. Spain became a natural forcing-ground for dance and dancers; it became a land for Spaniards, a land for dancing. It was impossible to escape its impact for it was everywhere present in convents, monasteries, churches, palaces, theatres, taverns, streets, patios and in the wide open squares, where everyone met everybody else. If people wished, they could all join in this dance pattern; it was part of the Spanish landscape and they had good reason to dance for joy. What nobody could forsee at the time was the effect this new form of dancing was going to exert upon dancing in the rest of Europe. Spanish dancing then, as now, excelled by its vitality; whether grave or gay, it was never dull nor was virtuosity lacking, even at that early date. It was like a richly-woven tapestry comprising oriental, occidental and nordic threads closely interwoven into the fabric of the solid homespun Spanish dances of the people—which has always remained the foundation.

The dancing masters perceived this and set to work with their creative fantasy to combine some of this new-found source of strength with the elegant formality of the court dances already in existence. Their foreign colleagues were not slow in copying them and the seventeenth-century suites of dances that were so prominent in the French *Ballets de Cour* bear testimony to the profound influence Spanish dance had exerted upon them.

Little was recorded in those days and evidence has to be sought in general literary, historical and musical sources in Spain. Only in the mid-seventeenth century was a method of teaching dancing to the Spaniards written down. Then, the steps were carefully codified into a system by Spanish dancing masters. Interest had been awakened in the subject of notation in and outside Spain. There was plenty of dance material to work on; the task was to classify it. This, the Spanish dancing masters set out to accomplish in the seventeenth century as will be seen in the next chapter.

4

The Growth of Spanish Dancing

THE SEVENTEENTH century was a period of tremendous literary, artistic and theatrical achievement. In Spain, the theatre prospered and therefore immense progress was made in this particular aspect of Spanish dance. That this progress was steadily maintained was due in a large measure to the efforts of the dancing masters, who were so active that the seventeenth century came to be known as the 'dancing masters' century'. Their task was simplified by the fact that suitable stages for dancing were laid in the new theatres then under construction. As more theatres were erected, most of the population acquired a taste for theatre-going. This applied not only to the capital but to the country as a whole.

The new structures called 'corrales' were a vast improvement on the fair booths, portable platforms and crude ambulatory theatres that had served in the past. The seventeenth-century corrales were specially designed as playhouses, erected on fixed sites and providing ample accommodation for a large audience. The two principal ones in Madrid were the Corral de la Cruz and the Corral del Príncipe (pl. 10), and it may be remarked in passing that the latter stood on the place now occupied by the Teatro Español.

A corral was in the open air, generally built in a square flanked by houses. The stage was erected against the walls of the houses, in such a way that a painted curtain could be attached to them and so serve as a setting for the entire play for as yet there was no scenery. In the audience, the sexes were segregated and a special enclosure called the 'cazuela'—literally 'stewpot'—was reserved for the ladies (pl. 11). Built on a slightly raised level from the ground floor, it faced the stage on the opposite side of the auditorium. The space reserved for the gentlemen was called the amphitheatre. Situated midway between the stage and the cazuela, it had separate entrances from the four staircases leading up to the ladies' quarters. Installed below the cazuela and almost level with the amphitheatre was the equivalent of a modern buffet, where the audience could go for a drink—a brew of honey, spice and water—or buy nuts, oranges and other delicacies.

Tenants on either side of the corral had only to open their windows to obtain a splendid view of the proceedings, but if other members of the audience wished to share these vantage-points, they had to pay an extra fee to the proprietor of the house, who reserved the right to hire his windows to whomsoever he chose. Tenants therefore had an alternative of paying to look out of their own windows, or admitting strangers into their homes during the hours of the performance. These rooms were much sought after by people who wanted to see the show without being seen and, above all, without having to make an entrance into the theatre itself. Small compartments with shutters that opened and closed at will, which might be considered to be the forerunners of present-day boxes, were arranged beneath the windows of the houses and they were generally reserved by members of upper and middle-class families (pl. 13). One of these was permanently booked for the municipal authorities and there was always one available for the king and queen, who enjoyed going to the corral together, or separately, incognito or disguised. All these boxes were provided with heavy curtains which could be drawn as desired, and in this way the occupants were not molested by the idle curiosity of the mob. Situated in the upper part of the corral were dim, gloomy compartments called 'tertulias' and these were occupied by monks, scholars or priests who could watch the performance in complete privacy, conveniently concealed behind the latticed windows (pl. 12). The general public thronged the central part of the theatre below. Placed immediately in front of the stage were benches, each seating three people, and a strong barricade separated these seated patrons from the others who, having paid very little, had to stand. No tickets were issued for this part of the house, but the rest of the public was obliged to pass through two doors, before they could enter the theatre and a fee was collected at each one. Payments made at the first door went to the author and the owner of the theatre. That at the second door was for entry to the theatre and a donation to the hospital—which was obligatory. Entrance to the cazuela had to be reserved and paid for in advance. Despite the fact that these theatres were primarily intended for the people, preference for reservation was always given to the aristocracy; a rich plebian could not have any seat a nobleman happened to want. Dramatists entered almost free and some tried to get in without paying anything at all and they were not the only gate-crashers. Guards had to be on duty to protect the unfortunate playbox attendants who apparently risked their lives when collecting the money.

Performances were given daily at 2 p.m. from October to April; at 3 p.m. in the spring and 4 p.m. in the summer. The doors opened at midday for the benefit of the patrons of the cazuela and amphitheatre. Anyone wanting front seats had to go early, for the first arrivals took the best places and only the very privileged could risk arriving at the last moment. To protect the audience from the hot Spanish sun, an awning was stretched across the auditorium in the summer and firmly attached to the houses on either side, and this is still customary in the Spanish open-air festivals. When it rained, performances were suspended, unlike today, when the orchestra and spectators have been known to sit in rain-sodden seats, while the dancers struggle with a wet, slithery stage (pl. 14).

According to Deleito y Pinuela's account of these seventeenth-century entertainments,[1] the turbulent crowds that hustle into bullfights and sports gatherings today are quiet by comparison with the average supporters of the corrales. Women adored going to the theatre; they lunched early, heard Mass and went straight on to the corral, where curious onlookers were already hanging around the entrances to watch the audience arrive. Once the ladies had found their places, they passed the time quite happily arguing amongst themselves, or called out to their friends in the body of the hall. Meanwhile, they munched titbits bought from the attendants who went round selling fruit, nuts, nougat, aniseed water and so forth,

[1]*Tambien se Divierte el Pueblo:* Madrid, 1944.

and their jaws never ceased to work. Neither did their tongues, as they chattered and laughed and, with ribald mirth, threw orange peel, nutshells or anything else that came to hand, at each other and at the men in the amphitheatre. These gentlemen sometimes bought delicacies from the attendants, making eyes at the girls as they received them and sometimes yelled remarks with bawdy humour. Isabel de Bourbon was not above frequenting the cazuela and on more than one occasion mischievously let loose reptiles, mice and other vermin to the horror of all present who, in their panic, gave vent to language scarcely fit for the ears of their queen.

Performances were advertised by means of posters placed at strategic positions outside the theatre, on the corners of houses, and in the most populous thoroughfares. These playbills were the first of their kind and were carefully written out by hand. They announced the time and place. Inside the theatre, the performance commenced with short blasts on a horn, followed by a parade of all the artists taking part in it, in the course of which the audience was politely requested, in verse, graciously to applaud in the appropriate places and kindly keep quiet the rest of the time. This preliminary was called a 'loa' and these loas were usually composed by someone other than the author of the play. After this introduction the audience settled down to enjoy whatever was being presented.

With an ever-growing theatre-going public, it was no easy matter to please everyone; the dramatists were at their wits' end to cater for all tastes and soon discovered that dancing helped. At first, the dances were purely incidental to the play, the public having to wait until the first interval before they could see the danced interlude, which was called an 'entremés' and consisted entirely of dancing. All the dancers taking part in the entremés were professional and their main object was to keep the audience amused while the actors changed their costumes for the next act. These dances were accompanied by songs, guitar, or perhaps a zither, and served a similar purpose as anti-masque in the English court masques. At the conclusion of the play, the dancers reappeared in a danced epilogue, usually comprising seguidillas or the daring and forbidden zarabanda. These dances were accompanied by castanets, timbrels and tambourines. The idea behind these danced epilogues was to send the audience home in happy mood. At the commencement of the century, the play was the most important part of the performance and dances merely incidental. They became so popular, however, that as time went by, they earned as much applause as the play itself; and then the authors began to use dances *in* the plays, adapting the dialogue to fit the mime, movement and gesture of the actors who confined themselves to simple little dances. If anything more elaborate were required, the professional dancers obliged.

The increasing use of professional dancers was one of the most interesting features in the development of stage dancing in Spain during the seventeenth century. Dancing acquired such importance that at one point the entire play became little more than a vehicle for the dances. Dramatists utilized Spanish dances lavishly in their works, principally to stimulate the action or to accentuate the dialogue; certainly not to show off the skill or grace of the executants. In their search for novelty, the playwrights exaggerated their use of dancing to such an extent that the authorities tried to put a stop to it altogether. In 1616 the council of Castille forbade all dancing in the theatre. It is recorded that 'as usual, the order was not carried out'. Those familiar with Spain will recognize this typical approach to authority. There were some people who defended dancing however; in *La Comedía de España* Casiano Pellicer wrote:[2] 'The dances cannot be abolished, for they are the spice of the comedies, which are worthless without them'. The dances were retained.

At a time when the themes of the plays were becoming more daring year by year, this surveillance of the dances before, during and after the plays, seemed incongruous. It may have had some bearing on the size of the audience. The open-air corrales were designed for a larger public, drawn from every walk of life; they were more spacious than they had been in the past and the dances occupied a more prominent place in the programme, therefore presenting a greater chance to demoralize a greater number of people, so it would appear, but this preoccupation by the authorities with the dancing contained in the plays indicates how important it was considered to be. Everything about the danced interludes became more impressive; the musical accompaniment was no

[2]*Comedia de España:* Madrid 1804; vol. 1, p. 132.

longer left in the hands of a couple of blind guitarrists. Bigger theatres and audiences required larger orchestras and viol, harp, trumpet and other brass instruments were added, as real concerts of music were given. With more elaborate music, more variety in the dances was possible; isolated dances became suites of dances, based on folk-dances as a rule and danced comedies, resembling little ballets, were produced. Inventiveness was not restricted to dance composition alone. The pieces were mainly of a lively, humorous nature and covered a wide range of subjects verging on the indecent at times. This was possibly what alarmed the authorities who traditionally were always on the look-out for immorality in the theatre.

Love was a favourite theme in the danced divertissements, not of a romantic 'ruins in moonlight' variety, but treated in more jocular vein. There were also burlesques of a simple, ingenuous, pastoral nature, in which set dances were utilized. The 'Lost Lover' was such a dance. The dancers crossed to change places, turned on one spot, crossed again to lose each other, and the dance concluded with a grand circle, facing in and then out. A somewhat pompous sounding title was 'The University of Love'; unfortunately no details were available as to how this idea was worked out.

Other much favoured subjects were those of topical interest, touching upon everyday life and bearing on politics. There was for example 'La Batalla' written by Navarrete y Ribera in 1640, depicting a naval battle in balletic form. Rattling castanets represented cannon balls; each dancer represented a ship; the men were Spanish, the women French. The Spanish ships were loaded with bars of gold while the French carried only trifling articles like flutes, bells, pins and syringes—with which to extract the Spanish gold.

Social satire was rife and dancing seemed to be one of the handiest means of expressing the people's thoughts. 'The Dancing School' was a comedy sketch, dealing with an ordinary dancing master, not attached to the court. It was by the same author as 'La Batalla' and caricatured the various classes of society in movement. To do this, the author introduced the reader to the master, the lackey who played the guitar for the lessons, and finally, the prospective pupils. They all implored the master to teach them a dance or two which he did. The dances he selected were intended to accord with their diverse stations in life. All of them were of the popular variety—canario, villano, sarabanda and folias, etc.

The canario had been called the 'father' of the jota in Spain. In those days it was a showy dance containing early zapateado steps. The step known as 'battuta del Canario' was a great favourite which resembled pushing the foot into a shoe and sharply tapping the ground with the heel, and may still be seen, arranged most beautifully and used in a most subtle manner in modern theatrical versions of the dance.

The villano, originally a peasant dance, consisted of movements performed on the floor as well as standing up, with the dancers clapping hands and slapping the soles of their feet.

The sarabande was also originally a folk-dance, said to be Spanish by descent, although there appears to be some doubt about the meaning of the word. When finally it was elevated to the court, it became known abroad as an aristocratic dance. This form of the dance was less well known in seventeenth-century Spain. A French visitor then remarked that the Spanish manner of dancing the sarabande differed from the French, but he did not enlarge upon the subject, or specify in what way it was different.

The folias was considered to be a wild, unruly sort of dance, usually associated with drunken crowds at village fairs at the period under review. Spaniards consider this to be Portuguese in origin, but it is very often danced in Spain in the streets, at moments of public rejoicing and on principal feast days. This dance was taken by the French dancing masters who developed it into a very elaborate social dance. Known as the 'Folies d'Espagne', it became one of the most fashionable, aristocratic dances of the period and was to be seen extensively in French court masques during the seventeenth century.

The seguidillas was frequently mentioned in Spanish plays. This was a dance that seemed ageless, for it cropped up in one form or another in every century. So profound was the influence of the seguidilla in the seventeenth century that Quiñones de Benavente was moved to claim in his play *El Murmurador* that all the latest dances were evolved from it. It was typical at that period to take dances of folk origin and include them in theatrical pieces, the idea being to add a flavour of local colour to the action of the play.

The people entrusted with the arrangement of dances were then obliged to seek new methods of presentation, and in this way countless new variations were invented. Other labels then had to be found for them, for it no longer sufficed to call them by their regional names; they had to be adapted to something of a functional nature, pertaining either to the occupations, industries or pastimes of the inhabitants or a certain neighbourhood. For example, there was 'Toros de Madrid' which combined dance movements with the faenas of the bullfight, apparently as popular a theme then as now for dancing. Another example was the pelota game, which incorporated the actions of the game with dancing, associated with the Basque country.

Abstract themes were not neglected either: 'Avarice and Liberty' or the 'Dance of the Fish and Wine' referred to the Lenten fast with contrasting movements to express the joys of eating meat again, once the fast was over. 'The Dance of the Harps', 'The Naval Armada', 'The Table of the World'—all these titles indicate something more than mere dance movements. Nowadays, they would conjure up a picture of something very akin to a balletic composition. So much for popular dances in the theatre.

The steady growth of dancing on the Spanish stage was not only confined to popular theatres. Those patronized by royalty were equally busy and the vast expenditure on masques and similar regal festivities was severely criticized on account of their extravagance. This was the period of court masques. In England we had the Merry Monarch, Charles II, on the throne with his 'Cuckolds all awry, the old dance of England'.[3] Dancing activity in France was fostered by Louis XIV, well known for his love of dancing and impersonating the sun. The splendour of the French *Ballets de Cour* was world famous. They were very formal in conception and considered to be the natural sequence to the spectacular balletic interludes, based on allegorical themes, that Catherine de Médicis

[3]Samuel Pepys (31 December 1662).

had introduced into France from Italy, in the hope of keeping her sons amused and thus prevent them from meddling in politics. And now what about Spain?

Philip III was on the throne at the beginning of the century and was a very fine dancer indeed. Too good, thought some of his entourage, spitefully remarking that he was better at dancing than anything else! Be that as it may, his reign was a pleasant one for the nobility. Dancing was an important adjunct to life at court and the royal entertainments provided a perfect outlet for it. They proved to be an ideal setting for the newly developed form of dance which the court indulged in, at times, so it was said, with too excessive zeal. The nobility were not content merely to act as spectators, but actively participated in the sumptuous theatrical performances given at the palace.

Any form of dancing improves with practice and the new elaborate style required not only practice but special preparation. Why, even the method of walking was so involved that it was believed that the assistance of a dancing master was necessary in order to master it! This kind of instruction was not confined to the court; even a gentleman of modest means could afford to have his children taught dancing. Dancing became an essential item in a girl's education and children at a tender age were expected to be instructed in this noble art. A seventeenth-century Spaniard laying any claim to being cultivated, was expected to know how to dance. Therefore, when it was decided to build a theatre adjoining the royal palace in Madrid, an appreciation for good dancing was already widespread among the vast Spanish nobility.

At that time, opulence represented authority to most people and masques were a useful adjunct to the elegant façade of court life; not only did they keep the courtiers amused, they also impressed visitors from abroad. Thus the political aspect of entertainment was not overlooked in Spain, and in form resembled that in other European courts. Professional pageant masters were engaged to supervize the productions, private theatres were attached to the noble houses and the best known among them were those attached to the royal domains. Many were within easy reach of the capital as, for example, El Pardo, Aranjuez, La Zarzuela, La Casa de Campo and La Granja. The most important of them all was in Madrid, at the Buen Retiro, now a public park.

It was Philip IV who commanded this theatre to be built adjoining the palace and bearing the same name. On 4 February 1640 the Buen Retiro Theatre was formally opened. The audiences attending the performances were the invited guests of the king when he was in residence. When he was not and the royal family was away, the theatre was open to a paying public. The Comtesse d'Aulnoy was sufficiently moved by the beauty of the interior to describe it in the following glowing terms in her *Voyage d'Espagne:* 'It is very lovely with paint and gilt. The boxes are provided with curtains like those at the Paris Opera House. In the royal box they are gold. Magnificent! Each box holds fifteen people; the Salon is quite large, embellished by lovely paintings and statues. There is neither orchestra nor amphitheatre, the public just sits on long benches.'

The long list of court entertainments, balls, banquets, masques, zambras, moriscas and various open-air functions of an original nature—all contained dancing in some form or other. The outdoor theatres were constructions of a temporary nature as a rule. They were built in the palace grounds which gave the gardens the appearance of an outdoors seventeenth-century drawing-room. When classical ballet production was added to the programme of royal gatherings, it was at the Buen Retiro Theatre that it was mounted in the grand manner. The Buen Retiro ballets were known for the lavishness of their transformation scenes (pls. 15, 16).

Stage designers, mechanics and technicians were brought from Italy to achieve these elaborate scenic effects, for in those days, the Italians had the reputation of possessing an ability for this, unknown elsewhere. As befitted an exclusive royal establishment, the auditorium was smaller than that found in a popular theatre, since it was intended to house only a small, select public. The stage opened out on to the garden at the back and when outdoor scenes were required, this was used as a natural setting, as scenes depicting love of nature were then coming into fashion. Three distinct sets were built in one production, each act with an appropriate set and even a different cast. The stage was crowded with people, passing and re-passing in a procession that resembled an army. Performances

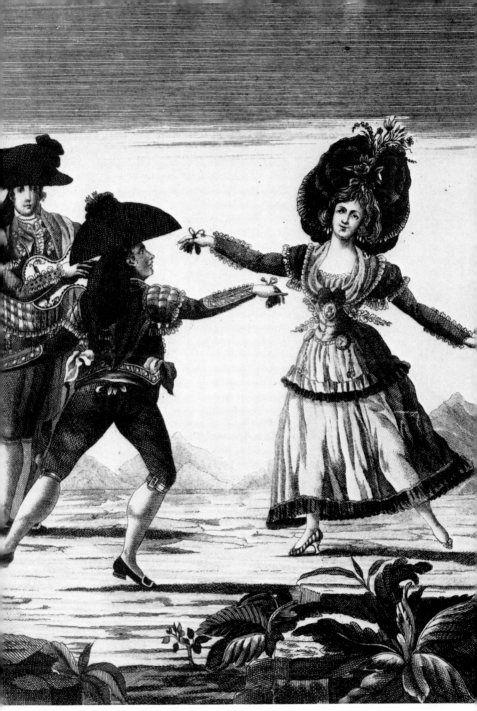

23. Eighteenth century bolero.

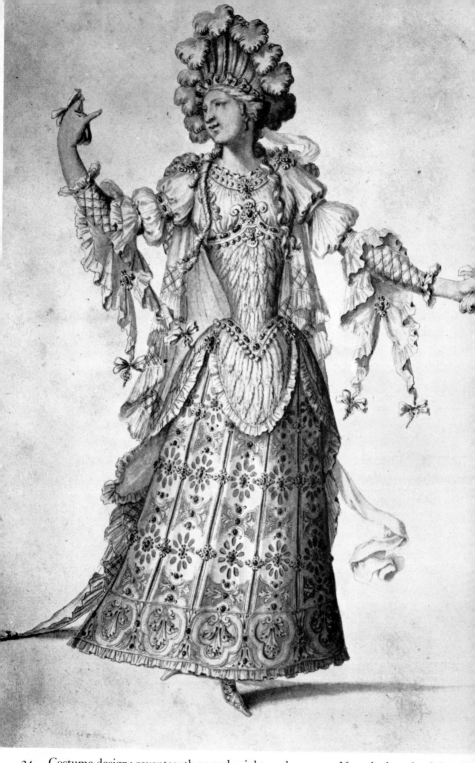

24. Costume design; seventeenth or early eighteenth century. Note the length of the ski

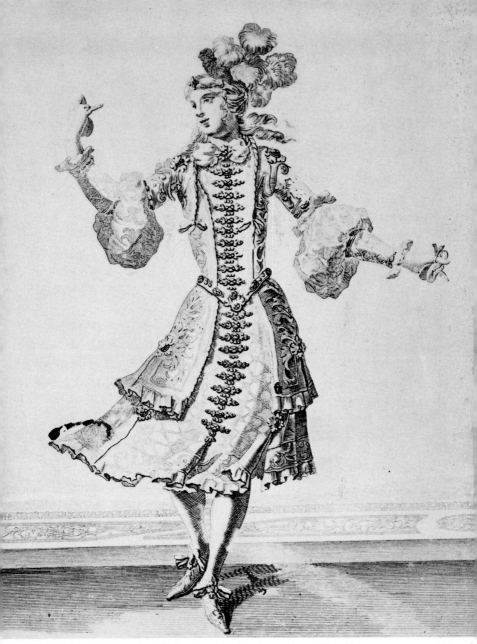

25.   Nymph in *Le Triomphe de l'Amour*. Note the shortening of the skirt.

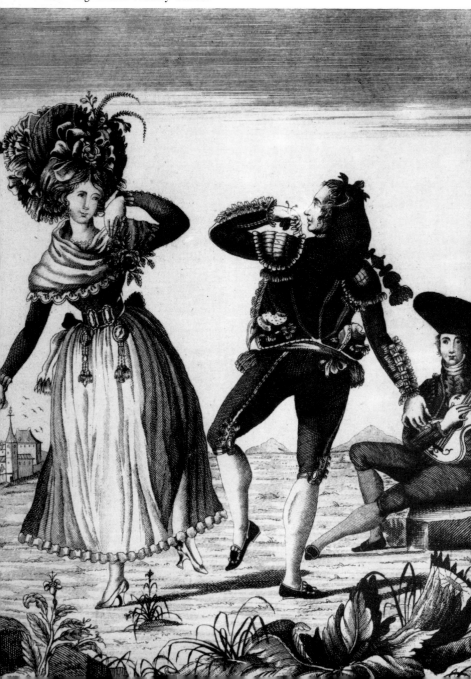

26. Eighteenth century bolero.

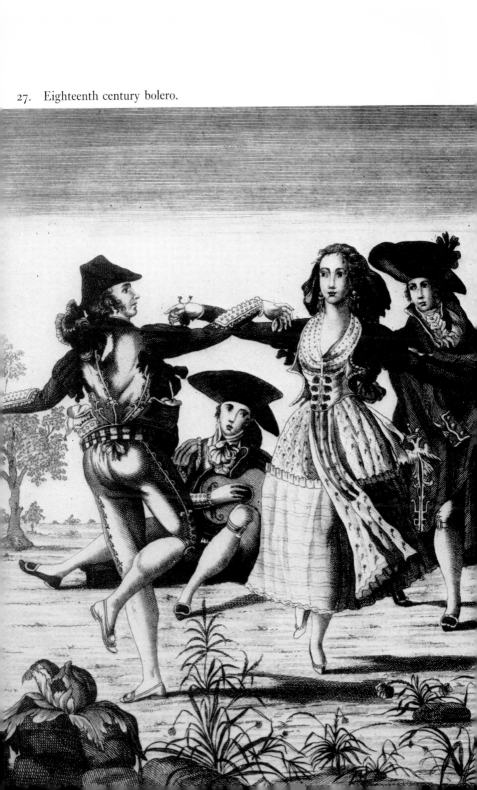

28. El Baile en San Antonio de la Flouda. From a painting by Goya.

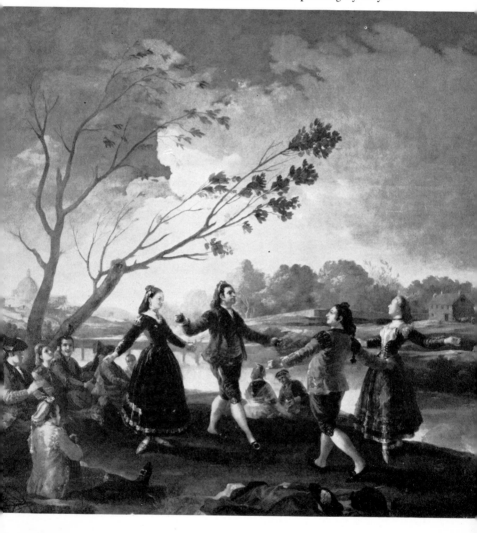

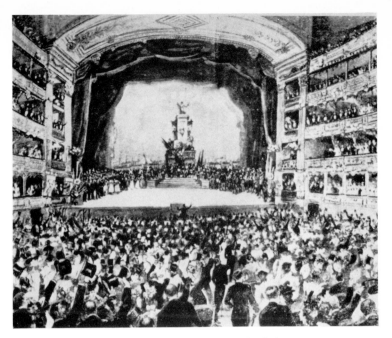

29. Interior of Teatro Real, 1898.

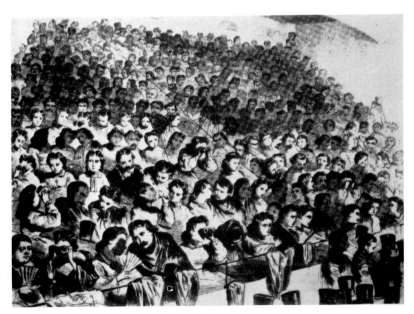

30. 'The Gods', Teatro Real, 1865.

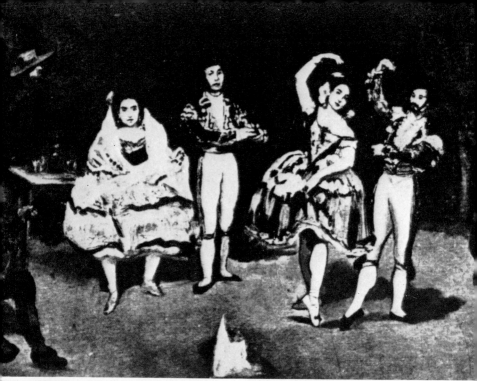

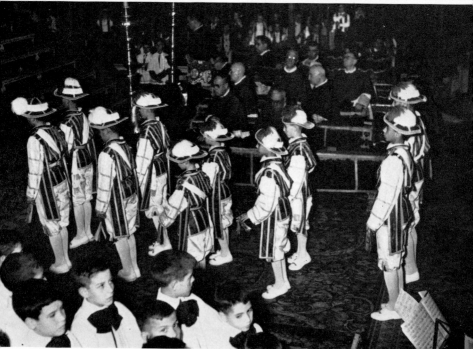

31. (*Upper*) Dolores Serral, an Andalusian dancer, famous for the cachucha.
She taught the dance to Fanny Elssler.
32. (*Lower*) Los Seises in Seville Cathedral.

in this theatre lasted for anything from four to six hours and during that time, drinks and other refreshments were served.

The outdoor ballets were no less elaborate. Some took the form of ballet-pantomimes and were held on the lake in the palace grounds. They were conceived on a majestic scale and in these, too, myths and legends were a favourite theme. The gods and goddesses, instead of coming down from heaven as they did in the indoor productions, sitting on their soft little clouds that went smartly up again at the appropriate moments, were aquatic deities, seated on thrones that glided along the lake, drawn by fish. They were encircled by naiads and tritons who sang and danced in the water—water was everywhere, it even spouted from the dancer's costumes.

No matter what the nature of these royal diversions, they all conformed to a type; a type consisting of a mixture of acting, singing and music, in addition to dancing, and the royal family often took part in them. The king, his brother, and the Infanta Maria Teresa were well known for their love of dancing and acting.

In 1649, the Infanta was complimented on her dancing of the españoleta (and was singled out for special praise)—not surprisingly. However, if she was a singularly hefty maiden, the dance she performed may have resembled 'Ye Españoleta' recorded in a manuscript to be found in the Bodleian Library, Oxford (Douce 280): 'Honour, take hands, fall into your pace, part with your pace, traverse sideways, meet with your pace and heave up ye woman in ye arms. Part againe, pace travers and meet againe; the woman, heave up ye man; honour and so end.'

In the following year, the Duc de Grammont went to Madrid to conclude the marriage arrangements between Louis XIV and this same Infanta, Maria Teresa. Other than the princess, the only thing that pleased him was the theatre he found there. Everything else failed to impress.[4] He wrote bitterly about the laziness and ignorance of the Spanish people which he found quite incredible—not only their ignorance of the arts and sciences but of everything outside Spain. In his opinion, a great deal of the poverty was due to the indolence of the people, the homes were only passably comfortable and in bad taste, as the Spanish had no taste in his opinion. The

[4]Duc de Grammont: *Diario;* National Library, Madrid.

three-hour concerts of chamber music provided to entertain him failed to do so and all he had to say about them was, that they might be all right for the Spaniards who were accustomed to that sort of thing, but to a Frenchman, they were diabolical! Nevertheless, he had the grace to admit that the laughter they provoked in his entourage was not in very good taste. The superb banquet in the Spanish manner, was likewise not up to French standards and brought forth the remark that neither he nor his retinue could eat the food! The only thing worse than the dinner was the concert they were forced to endure afterwards! Therefore, it was praise indeed when this critical visitor graciously admitted that the best thing he saw during his stay in Madrid was the theatre, which he found 'wholly admirable' and that he enjoyed the dances in the 'entreméses'[5] accompanied by harp and guitar, in which the dancers played castanets and wore tiny hats.

To mark the occasion of that marriage between the French king and the Infanta Maria Teresa, magnificent festivals were held on the Île de Faisans, a spot made famous by Cardinal Mazarin's pronouncement that 'Il n'y a plus de Pyrénées'. 'Pheasant Island' was situated on the frontier between France and Spain and Velasquez, the court painter, was sent there in advance of the royal party, to supervise the arrangements for the outstandingly beautiful wedding festivities that lasted for two months. They consisted of parades, tournaments, sailing in gilded barges to the strains of soft music, endless banquets and a succession of theatrical performances mounted on a scale difficult for us to visualize today. Of supreme interest to dancers, was the ballet that was produced in connection with this great occasion, appropriately entitled: *Il n'y a plus de Pyrénées*. This was a landmark in the history of Spanish ballet production and occupied just as important a place in the development of Spanish ballet as had the *Ballet Comique de la Reine* in French ballet production of the sixteenth century, the period in which ballet production in France steadily progressed, to reach its zenith during Louis XIV's reign (pl. 17).

Throughout the seventeenth century, so much was happening in

[5]'Entremés' were really miniature plays of a comic nature and at times they consisted entirely of dancing.

the realm of court-dancing, with monarchs on the thrones of France, England and Spain all known for their interest in dancing and each personally excelling in the performance of the dances then fashionable in their respective lands. In view of the advanced stage of dance development in Spain, it is interesting to conjecture how much of the progress of dancing in seventeenth-century France, particularly during Louis XIV's reign, was due to Spanish influence. His queen, Maria Teresa, was admired for her dancing. The finest dancing masters available were responsible for the ballets given at her wedding and no less a person than Velasquez had been entrusted with the artistic production. Historians dwell on the brilliance of the *Fêtes Nocturnes* held in France at Versailles. They were dazzled by their splendour, originality and cost. Less was heard about the actual source of the French dances. It should not be forgotten that in 1681 when *Le Triomphe de l'Amour* (pl. 25) was produced at Versailles before being transferred to Paris and handed over to professional dancers, a seven-year-old prodigy danced before the court, accompanying herself on the castanets and was much admired. One has only to look into later French records of the seventeenth-century masques to discover how extensively the French dancing masters drew upon Spanish dance material for their works. This being the case, it would seem that the matter is worth further investigation.

In the royal divertissements that took place at Versailles, playing the castanets while dancing seemed to be an indispensabls comple-ment to the dances. In Feuillet's version of 'Folies d'Espagne' he described not only steps but also the castanet beats. The section devoted to castanet notation he entitled: '*De la batterie des castag-nettes*'. Feuillet[6] used musical notes as symbols set on both sides of a line; those above referred to the sounds struck by the left hand, those below the line referred to the right hand. A minim indicated a roll on the castanets, a crotchet, a beat. Rolls on the castanets for both hands were included for left as well as right hands. This is quite a novelty nowadays, when a roll is usually performed with the right hand only—the left serving to beat the rhythm, as though in the bass. When a modern Spanish dancer was shown this seven-

[6]R. A. Feuillet: *Choréographie ou l'art de décrir la danse* (pls. 20, 21). 'De la batterie des castagnettes', p. 100. Paris 1701.

teenth-century foreign notation, she found it made no sense at all.

But let us return to Spain and the Buen Retiro Theatre, that worthy addition to the elegant splendour considered imperative in court life. Unlike the corrales, the royal theatre boasted a larger stage, fitted with every conceivable mechanical device then known to stage production. The right conditions were there to further the progress of classical ballet in Spain which was developing on similar lines to those in the rest of Europe at that time. The complicated scenic changes and fancy transformation scenes were far removed from the single set that had to suffice in corral productions. At the Buen Retiro, expense was no object and according to all accounts, the ballets stood out for their brilliance in already brilliant surroundings. Floods, fires, raging tempests and earthquakes were all vividly portrayed. The Spanish productions were not on such a grand scale as at Versailles; they were in a way, miniatures of similar functions. They also contained luxury and magnificence, but to a lesser degree; and the same type of spectacular diversion both in and out of doors. Nearly always, theatrical functions in Spain, whether popular or aristocratic, appeared to have possessed an individual, intimate note that was never completely obliterated, even in the most spectacular performances.

Mention must also be made of the dances included in the comedies presented at the Buen Retiro Theatre: 'Seguidillas de Eco', the jacara, canario, matachín, passacalla, menuetto and gallarda. All of them are figure dances and the danced interludes in these productions nearly always consisted of dances belonging to this group. For those interested in the actual construction of the dances, a small but informative collection may be consulted at the National Library, Madrid. They are described by the Spanish dancing master, Juan Antonio Jaque, and are thought to belong to the latter half of the century.[7] From this manuscript it will be seen that the Spaniards seemed to be very fond of figures that formed and reformed endlessly in various ways, half and full circles, danced clockwise or anti-clockwise, with quarter turns giving the impression of charmingly original shapes of a petal or scallop design in the

[7] J. A. Jaque: *Libro de Danzar de B. de Rojas Panteja.* Ms. National Library, Madrid.

ground patterns. The descriptions refer in particular to the jacara, villano and folias and give a very clear idea of the technical difficulty of the steps then demanded by the dancing masters. Once the simple peasant dances fell into their hands, they were simple no more. The turning steps alone would tax the technical prowess of any dancer today and there was a reason for this tendency to increase the difficulty of the steps. As dancing in the theatre steadily progressed, the dancers were forced to concentrate on the actual technical perfection in their performance of steps. This was particularly noticeable in the case of solo dancing. The insistence on the correct execution of steps marked a fundamental change in the outlook on dancing in Spain. The more important foot technique became, the more was specialized training demanded, and only a qualified teacher could give that. That was when the dancing masters came into their own.

The seventeenth-century dancing masters were most conscientious men and went to great pains to perfect their art. They worked continuously in an endeavour to invent new and better variations and competed with each other in their arduous task. They took enormous pride in their profession, made much money, particularly those attached to the noble establishments, and generally were highly respected members of society. They instructed their pupils in dancing academies or else privately in their own homes.

It was quite common at that period for dancing masters to write down what they taught and the Spaniards followed this custom. A most useful textbook for reference is that by Esquivel de Navarrho, who was attached to the court of Philip IV. Born in Seville, he studied with Antonio Almeda. This book entitled *Discourse on the Art of Dancing* makes his method of teaching quite clear and appeared in 1642. Contemporary with that of the celebrated French dancing master De Lauze, whose book had been dedicated to the rakish duke of Buckingham, Esquivel (1642) is in many ways complementary to De Lauze (1623) and stands between the Italian Caroso and the Frenchman. Esquivel agreed with De Lauze that the feet should be turned out, opposing Caroso, who taught that the feet should be straight.

In classical ballet technique 'turning out' the leg from the hip and bracing the thigh muscles has always caused a certain amount of difficulty to students, because this 'turn out' is an unnatural position. It is impossible to obtain a classical line without it and it forms the foundation of a balletic technique. This is why it is so interesting to find a Spanish dancing master insisting on 'turning out' at such an early date. In agreement with both Caroso and De Lauze, Esquivel also insisted on braced knees and these two technical details were indispensable fundamentals in his teaching. Describing the steps, he deplored the fact that too many dancers who had been trained in schools still did not know them. To rectify this deficiency, he gave a long list, together with minute instructions, as to how he wanted these steps to be performed and in which dances they were to be found. The text must be read with care in order to find out exactly what the master demanded, because some of the steps bear the same names as those taught by other dancing masters, but are not performed in the same way. The campanella for instance, as taught by Caroso, resembled the swinging of the clapper of a bell and developed into the balletic *battement en cloche* of today. Esquivel's campanella consisted of circling the feet, apparently round the circumference of a bell farthingale, which is more like a ballet *rond de jambe*. His teaching programme indicated what he expected his pupils to know: the alta, two variations of the pavane, six steps of the galliard, four variations of the folias, two of the rey, two of the villano, the chaconne, the rastro, the canario, the tordion, the pie de gibao, and the alleman. It is clear from this list that he taught both the court and the popular dances that had invaded the aristocratic ballrooms. Esquivel took the trouble to append a list of the leading teachers in Madrid and Seville, and also the finest executants of his day. Some of these people, incidentally, belonged to the most illustrious families in the Spanish nobility, which might suggest that at the time the best dancing was aristocratic. Obviously, dancing instruction of this kind in the seventeenth century represented as much an exact code of etiquette as it did a mode of dancing, for it reflected the exquisite courtesy for which the Spaniards were famous. As there was absolutely nothing instinctive about this kind of dancing, those who wished to excel in it were obliged to study long and seriously.

This was not the only aspect of dancing requiring specialized preparation either. That utilized in religious plays, processions and ceremonies had to be carefully rehearsed. In 1632, a man called Francisco Cerdau was engaged to teach the boys the dances that were to be performed at the Octave and Feast of Our Lady and he was expected to dance with them. For this he received 20,000 maravedies annually. In the seventeenth century, these performances were very prominent in the pattern of Spanish life. Religious culture was continued through this means and this practice was not confined to Continental Spain, for at that time the religious orders were very busy in the Spanish colonial empire.

What is so very interesting is to find that in this domain dancing was put on a professional basis. The dancers taking part in sacred plays and religious festivals were contracted annually, in much the same way as are choirs and organists today. In this matter, payment was graded in accordance with the type of dancing performed. Records show that the Cascabel dancers from Torrijos received only 1,700 maravedies whereas the Sword dancers from the same district were paid 3,000 maravedies[8] which looks as if Sword dancers were harder to come by.

No expense was spared in the preparation of these performances and a great deal of foresight went into their organization. Each character had to have a distinct costume and although we are not told who designed the costumes, a glance at the old expenses sheets reveals that they were worthy of any modern ballet wardrobe department. The fabrics were certainly not cheap; damask, taffetas, brocade are among them. A Turkish man and woman were dressed in blue damask; male and female giants in crimson damask, trimmed with gold and silver braid. A separate bill for haberdashery included white and coloured cottons, silver and coloured buttons, silver fringe, wax, cardboard and, funnily enough, 'wine for the officials'.

It was obvious that as dance production became more ambitious, help had to be sought from full-time professional dancers. In the case of the religious spectacles, although the dancers were paid for

[8]Coins made from copper and gold. Issued in the thirteenth century a 'maravedi' was worth about 25 centavos, that is, a quarter of a peseta.

their services, they had other occupations and were not necessarily what today might be termed full-time professional dancers; yet, when preparing for any elaborate religious celebration, they were anything but part-timers. The groups of boys attached to the cathedrals naturally worked on a full-time basis. They were taken when quite small, housed and fed and trained to dance and sing, in order to take part in the songs and dances included in the Mozarabe ritual. The kind of dancing connected with religious worship then, consisted of specially composed verses which the boys sang and then danced.

The only example remaining of this ancient ritual, may be seen at Seville cathedral where the Seises carry on the tradition (pl. 32). It is interesting to note that even this solemn dance form had a somewhat chequered career in the past. It was condemned for a time in the fifteenth century, when all dancing in churches, cemeteries, and religious processions was forbidden. It was in 1439 that a papal bull was issued finally permitting the Seises to dance before the high altar at Seville cathedral.

The 'Seises' was a name given to the boys because originally there were six; for some time now there have been ten, but the old title has been retained. They are reputed to wear the original dress and, according to legend, the Seises will continue for as long as the costumes last. Since this ancient institution is in receipt of an endowment, it is more probable that it will continue for as long as there are sufficient funds forthcoming to maintain it. The Seises in other cathedrals, notably Toledo, so I was told, had to be abandoned because what represented an ample sum for their upkeep in the seventeenth century, was no longer adequate.

The Seises were usually drawn from humble homes and had to be at least ten years old. It was not easy to become a Seis in the seventeenth century, for the aspirant had to be recommended by his parish priest or similar authority, who could vouch that there was no taint of illegitimacy in the family. It is recorded that, before being received for instruction at Toledo, a certificate had to be produced vouching for the purity of the child's blood—meaning, no Jewish or Moorish contacts. The dean had to be satisfied on this important point before the little boy could be accepted.[9]

As for the actual dance, it is a figure dance based on ground pattern, representing the figure of the Cross, symbol of sacrifice, sometimes taking the form of one large cross or splitting up into a series of smaller crosses; and the circle, symbol of eternity and the ancient serpentine pattern known as 'threading the needle' probably signifying wisdom. The boys enter in two parallel lines, reverently genuflecting, and slowly commence to dance, winding from one figure to the next and accompanying themselves on the castanets. Each dance figure is punctuated by a roll on the castanets and genuflection before the high altar. One verse is danced, the following one sung. Nowadays records may be obtained of this historical example. Once the voice broke, the boy in question retired and was replaced by a younger one.

This third type of dancing that must be added to the popular and aristocratic forms already mentioned earlier in the chapter, had one thing in common with the other two, and that was that it was first and foremost intended for public exhibition. The dances did not just happen, there was nothing spontaneous about them, they were worked out to fit into the framework of the ceremony or theatrical production, as the case might be. The dances were carefully rehearsed and the people taking part in them were paid for their services.

There is no doubt that the finest contribution made to the steady growth of seventeenth-century Spanish dancing was due to the efforts of the dancing masters. They went on without ceasing, developing old steps to make them more interesting visually and they also invented completely new ones. The chief interest was no longer centred on the figures or rhythmic patterns of the dances; steps claimed most of the attention, and as diversity in musical phrasing became general more elaborate sequences of these steps were evolved to fit the musical phrases. This all took place in the seventeenth century and the parallel development of musical and dance form led to real choreography. By the time the last quarter of the century was reached, the dancing masters were arranging steps into the sort of patterns that are still in use today.

⁹*Información de Seises:* Archivos históricos de Toledo. (National Library, Madrid).

The concentration of attention on the steps was an innovation affecting all types of dancing. This was in contrast with the past when Spanish dance form—or the outline of the dance—had been sharply defined, when the figures adhered to a set shape, but the steps were few in number and limited to those of the running and walking variety. Obviously, as steps became more varied and numerous, it began to matter how they were performed; emphasis was laid on their correct execution. There was a right and a wrong way of performing them and of fitting them into the ground patterns. Rhythmic construction, by reason of its diversity, became more complicated and the dancer either knew, or did not know, on which beat he had to start and, once started, how to time the steps. In other words, method was added to dance instruction. As more new and intricate sequences of steps were woven into the old dances, they became transformed at times into real feats of virtuosity. This factor more than any other distinguished Spanish dancing of this century from that of the past.

That less was heard abroad about these developments inside Spain was due no doubt to the fact that there was no organized school in Madrid similar to that opened at Paris in 1661 by Louis XIV, intended to train boys and girls professionally. Nevertheless, despite the lack of an officially sponsored academy, dancing thrived in the hands of the dancing masters, who did excellent work and made good use of it in the theatre.

Ballet production continued throughout the latter half of the seventeenth century at the Buen Retiro Theatre and continued well on into the eighteenth century, until Carlos III finally abandoned it in 1764. As continuous activity in other royal theatres also went on, the standard of dancing improved and ballet presentation followed along comparable lines with the rest of Europe at the same period. The day will have to come when somebody will turn his attention towards the study of the relationship of Spanish dancing in court theatres to that existing in the rest of Europe, notably in France. This should be done in order to determine the degree of Spanish influence exerted upon ballet abroad and especially on the famous *ballets de cour*, for these were the precursors of the *grands ballets d'action* which made such an impact on eighteenth-century production.

It was not by accident that in the seventeenth century, exquisite dances were being composed by the Spanish dancing masters. They were obliged to exert themselves in this direction as new theatres were constructed and more dancing was required in the pieces produced in them. If the dances were not to become deadly monotonous through being repetitive, the choreographers were obliged to seek a means of varying their arrangements. The growth of interest in theatrical dancing led to a demand for more solo dancing; this in turn required a certain type of execution and thus a taste for virtuoso dancing was born. As the steps evolved, Spanish dancing became very complicated and foot technique grew in importance. Specialized tuition was required and this the dancing masters provided; at times, they became positive dictators in the theatres, developing a renovated national style of dancing and producing some most interesting dance material in the process. Out of this, a synthesis of Spanish folk- and court-dancing developed. By the time they had successfully accomplished their task, external influences contained in the dancing of the past had been completely assimilated.

To sum up; the basic ground patterns remained simple; new steps were elaborated and old ones were added to them. Most important of all, it now mattered *how* they were performed. Positions were not yet clearly defined although they were slowly coming into being. Style was the primary consideration and this new style was, in reality, merely a continuation of the old sixteenth century school with its insistence on braced knees. Dances based on distinctive Spanish rhythms were now danced by everyone, not by one class alone. It was no longer necessary to look for the foreign elements contained in Spanish dance technique; the seventeenth-century problem was to recognize the native components within it. All thanks were due to the Spanish dancing masters who busied themselves with this matter and it was their systematic teaching that hastened the process of absorption. Little did they then know that out of the dance form they had developed, a Spanish classical tradition would emerge. They had laid the foundations for a method of teaching dancing to the Spaniards which, in the century to come, the Italians were to polish still further and develop into a universal 'school' or method of training that spread like wildfire through the opera houses of the world.

How this influenced the Spanish and foreign artists inside Spain as well as the growth of dancing in the theatre, will be considered in the chapters that follow.

5

The New 'Danceologies'

THE TRANSITION from Spanish to French court manners took place in Spain in the eighteenth century, when the Hapsburg dynasty ended and the reign of the Bourbons began. In 1701, the duke of Anjou, grandson of Louis XIV of France, ascended the Spanish throne and became Philip V. The new monarch did not speak Spanish and so French became the language at court. Where a Bourbon was on the throne, there a revival of interest in the arts was to be expected. Before long, French dances, as well as the French language, were the order of the day. The Spaniards were infuriated by the introduction of these unwelcome foreign institutions at first, but in time they adopted them and dancing in the French manner was accepted in the ballroom.

Dance journalism began to flower in Spain and many excellent textbooks on dancing were written in Spanish. They were not always well received. Moralists tended to dismiss them as diabolical, pedants regarded them with cynicism and many people treated them as a joke. The authors of the new 'dancing ologies' came in for their share of criticism and were volubly castigated in print by their colleagues. As dancing was converted into an exact science, certain scholars were inclined to sneer, loftily proclaiming that even the most insignificant things in life (meaning of course, dancing) could be treated scientifically—if one so wished.

All this opposition did not curtail the success of 'danceology' nor the sale of works on the subject. 'Ologies' in most things were modish at that time and, not surprisingly, dancing followed the general trend. In spite of the jeers levelled at this novel form of literature, some of the essays were quite serious in essence and throw an interesting sidelight on the position that dancing was beginning to hold in society. As will be seen presently, not all of the texts were written with malicious intent; some were clearly intended to instruct, and there were others obviously designed for amusement only. The profusion of such treatises suggests that the Spanish people were taking an ever-growing and intelligent interest in dancing of all kinds. Many of these productions were well larded with satirical allusions to French influence and were often concerned more with Francophobia than with Danceomania, but this may have been more a symptom of the acute nationalism that was then sweeping the country, than an indictment of the French manner of dancing. Spaniards then were as proud of their own traditional dances as they are today. They resented foreign intrusion in this domain, in the same way as they disliked the presence of the French in their country. Introducing French dances into Spain at that particular time served to heap fuel on to the fire of their burning nationalism. In view of this, it was miraculous that the dances survived, to gain ground as they did, until finally they were assimilated.

Spanish works at that period compared favourably with disquisitions of a similar nature written in other countries, about the same time. One of particular interest to dancers is that dealing with notation, choreography and the diverse manners of dancing. We will consider this first; then, secondly, a glib dissertation on the study of the contradanza; thirdly, a very Spanish document dealing with castanet playing; and finally, an original work dedicated apparently to impress upon the reader, the social pitfalls contained in too intensive a study of 'bolerology'.

The Spanish book on dance notation was published in Malaga in 1745 and entitled *Explicación de la Coreografía*. It was written by Boxeraus y Ferriol. Notation—that is, how to write down dances by means of visual symbols, was something that had yet to be learned. In this case, the positions and steps used in the fashionable dances of the period were described and particular attention was given to the contradanza. The Spanish manner of dancing was compared with foreign variations of this most popular dance that, for some time, had been sweeping through the ballrooms of Europe. Boxeraus was more interested in the arrangement of the steps than in how individual steps were performed. This choreographic aspect of dancing was quite distinct from that existing in the previous century when, as we have seen, the technical performance of steps mattered more than anything else to the dancing masters. In construction, this treatise was not unlike contemporary French works on the same subject. In many ways, Boxeraus followed the method for notating his dances used by the Frenchman, Feuillet, in 1699, although he allowed greater latitude in their interpretation than had his predecessor—in interpretation only, since the dances continued to adhere to a set form.

The contradanza was brought to Spain from France and it became most fashionable in the smart salons of the period. Despite the profoundly anti-French attitude prevailing in the country and the fact that many Spaniards were irritated by what they considered to be an effeminate, precious and affected form of dancing, the dancing masters did not let this sort of national prejudice trouble them. They not only taught the French version of the dance to Spaniards, they invented their own variations based upon it. Furthermore, they did a flourishing trade by writing down the musical scores and steps and selling them very cheaply—in time for the balls held at carnival time. The dance, complete with music, was written on a single sheet, all ready for the amateur to study at leisure at home without any aid from a teacher. This tendency to 'do it yourself' was very prevalent in the eighteenth century and vast quantities of these sheets were sold, which suggests that there was as great a demand for them as there was for similar notated instruction in other dances.

A perfect example of this type of pamphleteer was Pablo Minguet y Yrot who churned out with equal facility: *Dancing in the French and Spanish manner*, *Résumé of Reading and Writing*, *The Art of War*, *Meditation on the Sacrifice of the Holy Mass*, *A Guide to the Roads of Spain*—all of which were in addition to a whole series of booklets, telling people how to teach themselves at home in comfort and in their own time, the harp, guitar, and pretty well every other musical instrument. Conjuring was added to the list, for good measure.

The second type of book mentioned in our list is represented in his *Breves Explicaciónes de Diférentes Danzas y Contradanzas*. Minguet published this in 1765 and in it described minutely the arm movements, giving in addition many other useful tips to students. For instance, he advised short dancers to raise their arms to shoulder level, and taller ones, to keep them out of sight, down by their sides. He made the practical suggestion to those who found it difficult to remember the figures of the dance, to take a piece of chalk—or a stick of charcoal would do—then draw the figure of the dance on the floor and just follow the drawn design (a very theatrical device, still in use on the stage today, incidentally). Many of Minguet's designs were highly decorative, unusually inventive and were designed to help professional dance producers as well as the amateur dancer. One example for eight dancers showed no less than thirty different ground patterns which were very complicated (pl. 19). He suggested that if choreographers cared to vary the steps, these designs of his could be usefully adapted to theatrical dances, a suggestion which has been gratefully accepted by more than one contemporary dance producer when confronted with the task of grouping a large corps de ballet! These designs have proved of great value in arranging theatrical dances and a never-ending source of inspiration as they were obviously intended, not only for the salon, but also for the stage. This is not really surprising for it was quite usual to find social dances being adapted for theatrical use towards the end of the century. Figure arrangement formed the basis of choreographic works at that time and this fusion of social with stage dances became a salient feature of eighteenth century theatrical dancing. Before concluding this brief résumé of Minguet's work, one very ornate specimen of the contradanza should be mentioned. The title 'The Dandies' was probably intended to be a jibe at the French. Nevertheless, this, like many another French dance, became fashionable in Spain then and was enjoyed in much the same way as was French chocolate and Parisian millinary by those Spaniards laying any claim to be smart and up-to-date.

The next book on our list also deals with the contradanza, but treats it from a totally different angle altogether. This work does not appear to be intended either for the student or the choreographer,

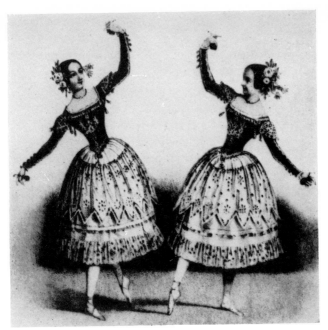

33. The famous Noblett sisters so admired by
Théophile Gautier.

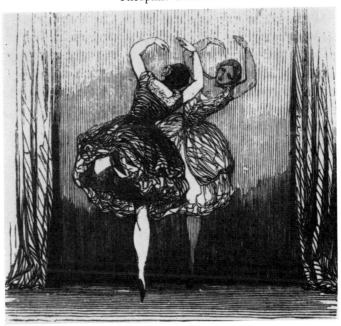

34. 'The Mirror Scene'. Marie–Guy Stephan.

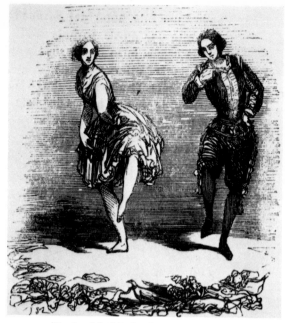

35. 'Farfarela'. Marie–Guy Stephan dressed
as a man in Travesty.

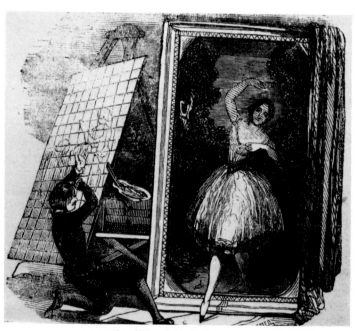

36. 'The Artist's Dream'.

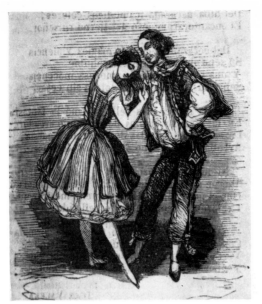

37. Marie–Guy Stephan and Marius Petipa.

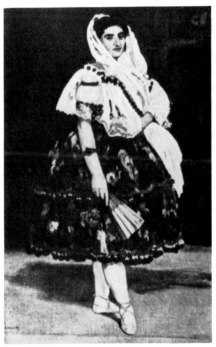

38. Lola de Valencia who taught Fanny
Elssler her famous cachucha. From a
painting by Manet.

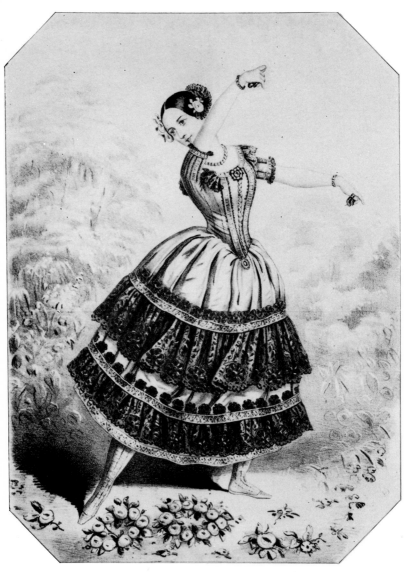

39. Fanny Elssler in 'La Cachucha'.

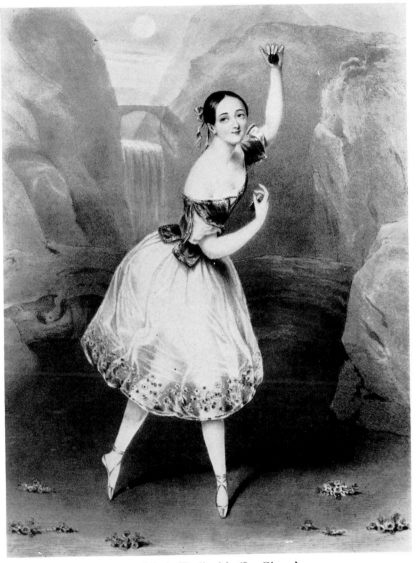

40. Marie Taglioni in 'La Gitana'.

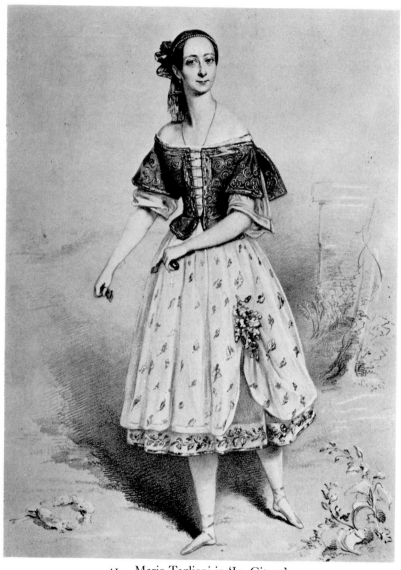

41. Marie Taglioni in 'La Gitana'.

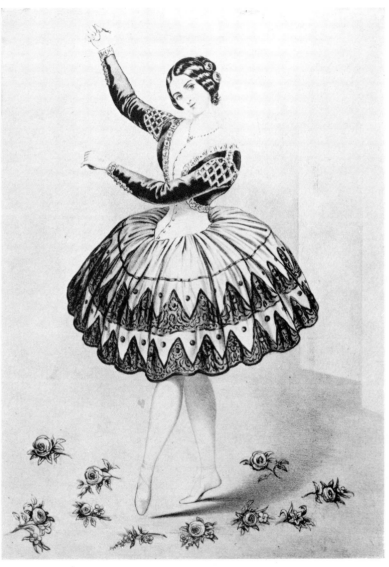

42. Lola Montes in 'Mariquita'.

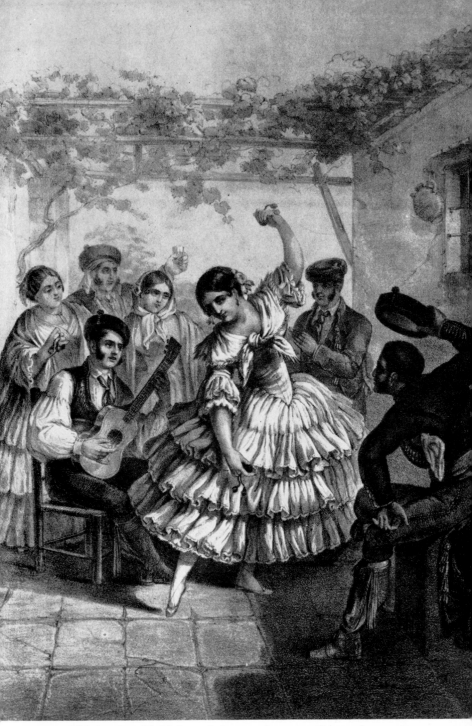

43. Girl dancing *El Ole* in typical open air surroundings; nineteenth century, probably Andalusian patio.

but it does convey to the reader the immense scorn felt by the loyal Spaniard for those foolish young people who were seduced by the charm of French dances. It is in fact, a printed condemnation of all who practise the contradanza. Written by a Basque lawyer bearing the pseudonym of Don Preciso, with the title *The History of Dancing and the Origin of the Contradanza*, it appeared in 1795. The book begins in an apparently lighthearted vein, gay and skittish, until suddenly, the author turns very sour and strikes with a viper's sting on his tongue—a tongue firmly in cheek it is true. First, constructing his 'science' and overpowered by moral scruples, Don Preciso proceeds to give his readers a dissertation on subjects far removed from dancing. There are two leading characters in his essay: Don Currutaco—a dude to the point of being a booby—is depicted 'arming' himself to go to the ball. He has a partner called 'Madamita' (little Madam)—a Franco-Spanish term intended to be facetious. In the early stages of the book, the author contents himself by joking about French contredanse and then suddenly pours out a vehement diatribe against this infamous foreign importation. A certain anxiety underlies his sarcasm; he senses in this alien form of dance, the dangerous influence it might exert on the youth of Spain. Don Preciso claims that the French evolved a 'science' out of the contredanse which the Spaniards only called the 'contradanza' because it was so completely contrary to anything they had ever known in dancing. Quite unlike Spanish dancing, it was so slight, it could be learned 'in less time than it takes to swallow an egg'. He proceeds to pour scorn upon the foolish Spanish youths who waste their time and energy on the dance. He takes quite a lot of trouble to enumerate the twenty essentials of his 'science' and throughout the book he continuously deplores the detrimental effect the contradanza is having upon the young people at court. His final pronouncement is that the youngsters are being thoroughly demoralized by studying the 'science' in the hope of reaping greater rewards through it, than by following their own occupations. A loud clarion call is sounded, warning them all of danger, exhorting them to give the contradanza a wide berth and mind their own business. Proud of Spanish national dress, he explains that most countries possess traditional costumes in which to dance, yet the supreme example is the Spanish majo dress, in which the bolero was danced. By comparison, the French dance was so poor that they had not even a decent dress to go with it! To remedy this defect and give further vent to his spleen, he recommends the 'little Madams' who are not too well provided by nature, to place a couple of small pillows inside their bodices or, failing these, a towel would do.

To deter the Spanish *jeunesse dorée* from going to their doom in the contradanza, Don Preciso prepared a little ballet synopsis for them, just to show them the depths that this 'dandies science' could plumb. It was entitled the *Hermáfroditas de Maxis* and was based on a mythical theme. Music issued from a cavern in the underworld, intended to accompany a contradanza performed there by the 'terrible god' Proserpine and the Furies—which just showed what a splendid dance it was. To strengthen his contention further, the author added that this particular form of the dance was not only French, but Anglo-French!

This intolerance of foreign dancing was by no means confined to Don Preciso and his set; it was widespread among the populace who then loathed everything French. In the realm of dancing, they showed their contempt by performing their own dances with renewed zeal, as much as a gesture of defiance towards the intruders as love of dancing for the sake of dancing. They paid homage to their land in a way they knew best by conserving the solid, home-spun dances of Spain and, at the same time, upholding their traditional manner of dancing. As a whole, the people avoided, whenever possible, all foreign dance products. It was the worldly set, inhabiting the capital, who thought it fashionable to embrace everything un-Spanish, because it must be more elegant and refined than their own, simply because it came from abroad. Not that they were any the less Spanish for that, they merely represented a type of person existing everywhere who is constantly running down his own country and customs, although firmly convinced of their inherent superiority.

The interesting point about this situation as far as dance development is concerned, was that these two strong nationalistic currents flowed side by side in the swelling tide of social dance and swept through eighteenth-century Spain. The vitality of Spanish folk-dance was gradually tempered by the balanced measure of French social dances and this fusion extended finally to all aspects of Spanish dancing.

We come now to the third book on our list, a strange work, entitled *Crotalogy, or the Science of playing the Castanets*. Published in 1791, it was written by an Augustinian living in a monastery in Madrid. His book is full of objections, also based on moral grounds, to this apparently harmless pastime. Castanet-playing seems a strange target for ironical wit, coming from a Spaniard, but at least the French were not held responsible—indeed Spanish dancers had been playing them for the past two thousand years! In the preface, the reverend gentleman claimed that his book contained an exact notion of the instruments called the castanets. Their origin, directions for use, together with the invention of harmonic castanets that could be tuned to blend with other instruments were all discussed. He reduced his precepts to a rigidly geometrical method. Shut away from the world, this satirical recluse was nevertheless obsessed by mathematical problems which he used as a means of venting his frustration upon the castanets. Violently sarcastic, even bombastic, the book is fascinating by reason of the amount of attention given to such an apparently innocent victim as a pair of castanets. It begins with: 'Supposing that they are to be played, better play them well than badly.' A collection of definitions, corollaries, articles, canons and axioms follows and the treatise ends up with: 'Mature men have always grumbled and scolded when offended by the noise of harmonious castanets, but youth, mad as ever, is always attracted by luxury, noise, feasting and amusement as a legitimate vehicle for indecency.'

This author, like Don Preciso, takes the opportunity to taunt the fashionable world for its obsession with foreign articles. In Article 4, a corollary states that because of their beauty, box, pomegranate and similar woods were highly suitable for making castanets but suffered from the grave defect of being found everywhere in Spain! For this reason alone, mahogany, sandalwood, or better still, ivory were preferable, for they possessed that highly desirable whiff of foreign lands, so indispensable if they were to be recommended to people with any taste. Canon 1 lays down therefore that, although

Spanish wood produces the same effect as foreign wood, it is no good for castanets. To attract attention, castanets must have some peculiarity in colour or manufacture—it may be necessary even to order them from Paris and, to achieve this end, neither diligence nor expense should be spared. Canon 3 states that ladies in particular should take care to match the colour of their castanets to their own individual type of beauty. A blonde should use ebony and a brunette, ivory; for the sake of symmetry, the cords attaching them to the fingers must have a set number of strands—fixed by law. It is a crime of 'lèse-crotalogy' for dancers to appear with ribbons the same colour as their shoes, hairnets and other paraphernalia that serves to keep the hair in place. Exception: gold and silver trimmings go well with all colours and castanets.

Observation 2, part 1, section 1: 'Daily seeking knowledge hidden from the rest of us, the tireless efforts of scholars have resulted in the discovery of something we all knew—that there are poplars. But what we did not know was that they married and had wives. We now know that there are male and female poplars, male and female plum trees and female oak trees. In this way, modern thinkers have discovered that in castanets there is also a diversity of sex— male and female castanets—but, in spite of all the anatomy that I have done and all the microscopes I have looked through, I found no difference, but I do realize that such differences are always more clearly revealed to the lucky idiot than to a laborious scholar.

Theorem: 'Being of common opinion and without bothering about further proof, a male castanet contains more wood and is therefore thicker and more sonorous than the female, which is slimmer, sharper and more subtle. We are eruditely informed in a paper of the 19 November, that one of the distinctive features of the male voice is its depth and that of a female voice its thinness, so it is with castanets. Q.E.D.'

Ponderous though this satire is at times, it is interesting in that it shows that people were as intrigued then, by this most necessary complement to Spanish dancing, as they are now. Foreigners still want to know when it was that Spaniards first began to accompany their dances with castanets. To answer their question we have to refer to the early works on 'crotalogy'. Crotalogy was a term used to define the art of playing the castanets, in literature of the seventeenth and eighteenth centuries. Their origin is of considerable interest.

From books based on early records, we learn that the women of ancient Egypt not only played with them, they also used crotalos as ornaments. They consisted then, of concave pieces joined together with ribbon and were worn in pairs. The priests of Egypt, when they went to make sacrifices before the altars, were preceded by maidens with crotalos in both hands. The girls marked the beat of the pagan dances with them. Women warriors in Hannibal's army went into battle to the sound of crotalos. Roman women attended festivals, wearing large flat pearls with holes pierced at the top, through which ribbons were threaded for it was then considered that the sound of these pretty little ornaments gave added charm, even coquetry to their movements as they walked. The crotalos both from Rome and Egypt were made from diverse woods and metals, or ivory; they were oval in shape, concave with a protuberance at the top, like a tiny ear.

Some of the earliest Spanish dancers we know who used crotalos were the famous dancers of Cadiz, and the contemporary writers who recorded their performances were impressed by the noise these instruments made as the girls danced.

Today, there are many types of castanets and their resonance depends upon their size and weight. Some are high pitched, others are quite deep in tone. The light ones are usually played by girls and are generally smaller than those used by men. When played in unison, the tone is better if all the dancers use castanets made from the same material, such as wood, plastic, or metal, whether they are to be played by men or women, but for solo dancing, uniformity of tone is not so important. The sound of castanets can be very pleasant to the ear when produced by four pieces of wood of the same size. The tone should be even, dry and shrill, except when the effect of a roll is desired, when it should exert the same soothing effect upon the listener's ear as that of the human voice executing a perfect trill; even and soft, with the underlying rhythm clearly defined by the bass castanet which is held in the left hand (pl. 22).

To return to the eighteenth century and the last book on our list.

The most favoured Spanish dance was the bolero, especially during the reign of Carol III (1759–88). The bolero was the Spanish answer to the French contredanse. It was a favourite dance in the ballroom and every young Spanish girl was expected to know it. Not only a dance, it later grew into a 'school' and qualified for an 'ology'. *La Bolerología* was written by Juan Jacinto Rodriguez. In it, he drew a very fine picture of the bolero dancing schools as they existed in Madrid in 1795. He dedicated it to 'the knowledgeable pupils of the bolerological academies in Madrid, Cadiz, Seville, Cordova, Murcia and all other towns where bolero schools existed'. Here again we are warned against the dangers of the dance, even a Spanish dance, yet this writer was no priest. He observed: 'Their [the dancers'] great souls, not content with ordinary festive dancing, yearn for something demanding skill, agility and the management of the body. Preachers may reprove the dancers, warning them that such dances are leading them straight to Hell. It does not make the slightest difference to them if these mentors grumble, scold and yell. For what matters most is what these dancers like and, the better their legs, the sooner the demons will take them.' (pl. 26.)

Perhaps this sounds a little harsh but the first part of the book helps to explain this reaction. A sub-title announces 'Anti-Bolerología or, the Total Ruin of Dancing'. An interesting description of an eighteenth-century dancing academy follows. The academy was situated in the house of Signor Caldereta in the Calle Ballesta where, every evening, he gave his lessons. The visitor had some difficulty in gaining admittance. Knocking twice and receiving no answer, he was obliged to batter loudly on the door with his sword. That brought an old lady dressed in majo costume who, before opening it, wanted to know who was there. She insisted upon being fully reassured as to his identity before she would consent to let him in. On entering, he observed that the room was quite spacious, that the walls were adorned with pictures depicting signs, symbols and figures relating to the 'science' taught there, but they were so blackened that the original painting could scarcely be seen. Long benches served to seat the spectators. From the grimy ceiling were hung twenty or thirty ropes that might have been used to hang bacon and 'the strangest things were done with them'. There seemed to be about a hundred and twenty people there, apparently all novices and of such diverse shapes and sizes, that it made one think 'that our Spain abounds in madmen . . . . Dense smoke from lighted cigars permeated the eyes, nostrils and mouth, and had I not been used to it there is no doubt that I would have been smothered. The Maestro approached, made a graceful bow and after greeting me "a lo Jerezano", invited me to take a seat, as he must start his class.'

The visitor proceeded to give his impressions of the classes:

Tuning his guitar, he, the master, ordered the pupils to begin by loosening up, whereupon the battle began and, to put it mildly, all hell was let loose. Some grasped the ropes hanging from the ceiling and, supported by them, began to practise cabrioles, whilst others did their steps round the room, performing a thousand variations. With no deference to modesty, some of the women lifted their skirts above their knees, so that their positions could be seen more clearly, meanwhile leaning on the shoulders of the boys who lifted them, then put them down again. Trying to do turning steps, the skirts flew over their heads and, had it not been for the white, close-fitting pantaloons they wore, something that respect and modesty prevents me from mentioning, would have been seen! Abandon, immodesty and prostitution powerfully attract hallucinated youth, who thoughtlessly embrace the worst forms of depravity, thereby forsaking the decorum and reserve fostered by a good education. What could I do? Since the dance was about to start, I could not very well leave the room. Horrified by what met my eyes, I turned to converse with an elderly lady seated beside me, enquiring if she danced? 'No, sir,' she said, 'I have been suffering from a chest complaint for the past few months, which has prevented me from dancing but, although I say it myself, I have a daughter who is the best bolero dancer at court.' 'Is your erudite daughter here?' I asked. 'No sir, I pay twice the price so that she may study privately in another room. If you really knew what you were talking about, you would realize that without a complete knowledge of the bolero, nobody is completely educated. One must be able to dance two or three variations, no matter how, good, bad or indifferent. Unfortunately for me, I was born at a time when only a passepied or an aimable was danced and the ordinary people did a ridiculous fandango.

This eighteenth-century 'dancing Mamma' goes on in the same strain, explaining that she has a professor to teach her in spite of her age, but too much exercise has given her an affliction of the chest that prevents her from playing the castanets. Her daughter, therefore, would have to perpetuate her memory by excelling in the performance of the bolero. The girl was also learning the 'fortpiano' and French. With these accomplishments, she was receiving a really fashionable education which would equip her to take her place in any society. There were plenty of admirers already. Only a few nights ago, a certain count was heard to remark that he would never marry a girl who did not know the bolero, which was a most elegant and patrician dance (pl. 27).

By now, the dancers were sweating, which resulted in a fetid odour, enough to make even the most hardened gravedigger reel! Dense smoke puffed from more than sixty lighted cigars, permeated the room as though emanating from cellars or coal holes. The ever solicitous Maestro Caldereta, darted about to correct his pupils' dancing. Dona Clara appeared, rattling her castanets, faced the doughnut-seller, who signalled the guitarrists to strike up a copla of the seguidillas on his half-tuned guitar. The daughter's skill was greeted with thunderous applause and thinking, she might give a second demonstration of her bolerological ability, she succeeded in putting herself out of action before the end of the dance—and, incidentally, for the rest of her life! Such acclamation had been too much for our ballerina who, trying to surpass herself to the extent of tackling an entrechat six, twisted her foot. She fell on to the left foot with all the weight of her body and this broke it. The formidable noise of the castanets ceased and the only sound to be heard were the screams of the unhappy girl. Her mother smothered her with kisses, drowning her unfortunate daughter in a torrent of tears, whose cries only subsided when she fainted away. An unhappy victim of bolerological fanaticism, she came round emitting shrill screams, imploring her mother to take her away from the place . . . .

A vivid caricature indeed of an unhappy victim dedicated to the bolero. The author does not confine himself to the dancers but goes on to treat the actual steps with the same scornful derision. Dancers, and ballet students in particular, will be entertained by the original slant given to some of the eighteenth-century definitions to many steps still used in classical ballet. For example:

'Glisá' today is called a 'glissade' and looks very graceful, like weaving the feet in and out, and it is not difficult to do. Cadiz was its birthplace and an adjutant of the Engineers Corps called Don Lobara Chinchilla invented it. The heroic professor is said to have called it 'Glisá' because it was derived from 'glasus' meaning a kind of fortification, as he had the intention of leaving it to posterity.

'Pasura' resembles a *pas de bourrée* and is used a lot in the bolero. This movement really consists of two in one and was discovered by Pereta Zarazan, native of Ceuta and possessed of greater mind than fortune. After practising bolerological exercises for two months, he broke a leg and died peacefully, surrounded by his co-citizens.

'El Taconéo' is heel tapping and stamping. What symmetrical noise is heard when this movement is performed! The heel is shown to advantage in this step and dancers deserve loud applause—even from the ignorant folk present. According to our knowledgeable secretary, Pitti-Coloni, a Mallorcan shoemaker, invented it to stimulate trade and introduced it into Spain where it was first exercised in Cartagena. 'Paso marcial', ye gods! You mean to say that there are military evolutions in the bolero?' 'Yes, sir, there are, and this is not the only one, for you see something of all the others is embraced in our bolerological science.' The Paso marcial is the work of Rudolfo Engama, sergeant of pensioners from Almeria. This good man, having developed a cough, continued to practise bolerologia too much and found it necessary to apply for retirement. In view of his uselessness this was easily obtained. God bless my soul! [The bolero was useful even to a blue cap and white belt.]

'Advance and Retreat'. This name is purely and simply military. 'Puntas or Pointes'. Grotesque positions that deserve general applause when well executed. The feet are placed in such a way that it seems that the dancers intend to fly. Moreno the famous professor who reached the summit of bolerological science invented this, and his name ought to be written in letters of gold to his eternal memory.

'Vuelta de Pecho'. Here, now, is where the skill and agility of good dancers are to be recognized, for one needs inordinate lightness to do this step. Eusebio Moriles was the author, a banister-maker from Alcara de Henares, who left his job to embrace this admirable science. He died from haemorrhage started by this invention. Many followed in his footsteps and, according to the latest news, it has thrown more people into the next world than the Lisbon earthquake.

'Vuelta perdida'. This was the name given to a movement that finished with a turn. There is nothing difficult or dangerous about it, which is its greatest recommendation. Only once did a certain professor dislocate his right foot doing it, and it is unnecessary to mention his name but the name of the inventor. Yes, for he exercised bolerology during three consecutive years in Madrid, with the greatest possible success, until the jealousy of his contemporaries obliged him to seek refuge in Cordova. He was called Don Curaco Galliedo, native of Valladolid in Castille, and his profession was doctor, or matachin.

'Trenzados with 3, 4, 5 and 6'. These are beats of the entrechat family. Many things are understood by a single word as can be seen by the word 'trenzado'. It is in these steps that dancers of both sexes can best display their ability and in which girls in particular can show off. It is unthinkable that they wear long 'pantaloons' and skirts, because if their calves can't be seen, there is no point in their performing these different beats. El Bolero has its own special dress, which has been, and is for all time, that of the maja. The supreme Bolerological Assembly forbids, on pain of notorious impropriety, that individuals, either male or female, should appear in long skirts, either in theatres or on stages in European or colonial territory. The inventor, now a performer at the Barcelona Opera, a studious man, although Venetian, idolized Spanish dancing and published a catalogue of seguidillas that many people pretend were unknown. Anyway, Lazaroni, as this Venetian was called, became famous through his Trenzados.

'Bien Parado'. The whole bolerological science lies on the 'bien parado'. Yes sir! The dancer who does not know how to stop gracefully and rhythmically, does not deserve any applause, no matter how exquisitely he performs. As a result of representations made by all the bolero masters, the 'bien parado' becomes a subject of daily debate. One thing is decided today, another tomorrow; today one is allowed to stop in the third position with the feet placed together; tomorrow, it is decreed that the left foot remains in the air as a preparation for the jump. An edict is issued admonishing dancers to return the arms to the natural position by their sides when they stop, when already there is another proclamation allowing arms to be raised symmetrically. The touchstone of all bolerology is the 'bien parado'; the same is true of the 'paseo', when the partners cross to change places. Ever since Antonio Boliche stylized twenty or thirty different ways of doing it, it varies daily, but going here or there is much the same always and the only variation is in the name.

The bolero has now extended throughout the universe and there are few countries that do not know and admire it. Sweden is particularly addicted to this dance, and in Stockholm apologies for bolerological exercises in a cold climate have been published. The Russians, following the good taste of their neighbours, the Swedes, have set up the first school in the North. Here, there are actually Lapps, Tartars, Poles and other sorts of 'birds', and most expert professors are to be found in these two attractive parts of Europe. In parenthesis, it may be noted that the word 'bird' is sometimes used in Spanish to denote an effeminate man. Nearly all foreigners give the bolero another name, but there is only one dance called the bolero, and Spain quite rightly boasts that she is the true mother of the dance and Spaniards are the finest bolerologists in the world. Throughout the Peninsula, whether in new or old Castille, Aragon, Valencia, Murcia, or Andalucia, a young person's education can be gauged at once by what he knows about bolerology. To be a useful member of society, we believe that every citizen should have some idea of the bolero and what it is.

This extract makes it quite clear that at the end of the eighteenth century, the bolero was in the forefront of Spanish social dances, even superseding French dances in public favour. The Spanish people, by then, were obviously no longer so impressed by foreign 'ologies' and other manias engendered by dancing, as they had been formerly. Nor were they impressed by dancing that was exaggerated, or practised for ulterior motives. The references to the snobbery, vanity and affectation hitherto usually associated with dances from abroad was now applied to Spanish dancing. The traditional Spanish criticism that dancing is morally perverse might be expected—indeed, seemed inevitable. What is unusually interesting is to find in this kind of book, so much technical information emerging, concerning how the feet were placed; the tendency to rise higher on the ball of the foot and the increasing use of beating, turning and springing steps. The critics then, might find it odd that dancers should bother about such details as whether their arms were over their heads or down by their sides or if the positions of their feet were open or closed, but the fact that they noticed this disparity in these matters would suggest that the absolute dictatorship so peculiar to the seventeenth-century dancing masters no longer held, and the dancers could now choose for themselves what they cared to do.

The Spaniards were not averse to criticizing the misuse of their very own bolero but never for one moment did they forget—or allow others to forget it either—that this was a national dance and therefore had to be taken seriously and never be allowed to be burlesqued. When this happened, they became their own severest critics.

The bolero is so important in the history of Spanish dance, that the time has come to define it. Not only was it the name given to a dance, it was a term also applied to a method of training used to prepare for a certain type of stage-dancing called: 'The Classical Bolero School'. Any executant or teacher in this branch of professional dancing was known as a bolero or bolera. Since this was no ordinary kind of dancing, the dancers specializing in this type of Spanish dance must not be confused with the common or garden bailador. Old programmes make it very clear what the position was; there were first and second ballerinas, first and second boleras, first and second grotescos. These titles all indicated what these dancers were engaged to do in the theatre.

The bolero, as a dance, was as conspicuous in the eighteenth-century ballroom as it was on the stage. Boleros were also frequently to be found in the second danced interludes of the operas and then had special names, such as 'The Smugglers' Bolero', 'The Bolero of Liberty', 'The Chocolate Bolero', 'Bolero of Carlos III', according to the subject of the piece. The system of naming boleros after famous individuals became very fashionable, a fashion lasting well on into the nineteenth century. 'Olé de la Curra' was so called after a famous dancer 'La Curra' who lived in the early days of the century (pl. 23).

If the origin of the dance is obscure, that of the word bolero is still more so. Learned Spanish authorities do not always agree on this matter. One theory is that in the eighteenth century, the famous dancer Ceresa visited his native village and saw the lads of the village dancing with such ease and elevation that they appeared to fly; *a volar*, means in Spanish 'to fly' and this was corrupted to 'a bolero'. Ceresa came from La Mancha, the home of the seguidillas and it is said that he invented the dance about 1750. Another theory is that Seville was the home of the bolero and that Antonio Boliche of Seville was the man responsible for it. Whatever uncertainty there may be about its birthplace, one can be quite sure about one thing wherever it came from, and that is that it passed through many stages of development before it reached the theatre and the ballroom.

Little did the 'Dancing Mamma' at the bolerological academy realize, as she scornfully dismissed the 'common fandango' because it was danced by the people, that the bolero too started life as a popular dance—in common with many dances at that period that graduated from the village square to the ballroom. Only when boleros came to court did they become polished and refined and subsequently, fashionable among the élite. It may be remembered that William Beckford expressed surprise that hardly any floors were boarded in Madrid in his day, and he remarked that the custom of dancing on rugs was universally established. That alone would serve to modify the movements of any folk-dance. As for the theatrical version, by the time the bolero reached the theatrical stage, it had become a most brilliant exhibition of highly developed, difficult steps. The Italian dancing masters were responsible for this, as they superimposed Italian technique upon the old seguidillas, adding to this ancient dance form, jumped, beaten and flying steps and delightful adornments in the use of the arms.

Musically, the bolero is in triple time and played at a moderate speed. It was usually accompanied by guitar, castanets and drums.

In the popular version of the bolero, the dancers originally danced four coplas. A copla consisted of thirty-two bars of music and there was a pause between each copla to give the dancers breathing space. In this form, the dance was collective and the steps were traditional, but if the dancers were clever enough there was nothing to prevent them from improvising upon them if they wished. This practice was not confined to Spanish dancing, but was commonly found in most popular forms of dancing everywhere at the same period. The bolero was used in many different ways, once it was transplanted into the theatre; it could be a solo, or for two, or three, or more dancers. As a solo dance, it became very intricate as the dancer could show off anything he or she was particularly good at—and there was plenty to choose from, in the endless sequence of jetés, assemblés, glissades, sissones, *pas de bourrées*, pirouettes and beats. Light, stamping steps were allowed, but nothing heavy or coarse. The pause was eliminated and the dance flowed on smoothly, without a break. The introduction of big jumping steps created a great sensation, as great as the shortened skirts which became more than ever necessary, as the variations became more brilliant.

Even in the more elegant social form of the dance, the bolero demanded great virtuosity, since it was invariably accompanied by the dancer with castanets; as for the stage version, to be really proficient at it, the dancers had to submit to arduous, systematic training, for much of its effect depended upon sheer technical strength. Despite this, there is no evidence to show that the theatrical version of the dance ever degenerated into acrobatic fireworks, as had other social dances once they were made into stage dances. Spanish classical dancing of the Bolero School possessed as it does today the refinement of eighteenth-century academic dancing; elegance was and remains the hallmark of this most distinguished form of dancing. Perhaps it is this quality that attracts so many ballets students to it everywhere, nowadays.

The reason why it has been necessary to deal with the bolero at some length, is that no other single Spanish dance made so great an impact upon every other type of dancing in Spain during the eighteenth century. Many Spaniards considered 'bolerology' to be a joke chiefly because it was not customary to regard any dancing in the light of an 'ology'—and least of all the Spanish bolero. This mental attitude was imported from abroad.

Originally a dance of the people, the bolero might be expected to retain its popularity; after all it was what happened to most folk-dances at that period. That it became a mania in the ballroom seems surprising but is explicable, taken and used as it was, as a bulwark against foreign intrusion, which threatened to swamp the Spanish social dances then in fashion. The ballroom bolero was the Spanish answer to the challenge of the French contredanse. What is not so clear, is why a national dance like the bolero, did not go the same way as the jota and fandango, which remained in the hands of the people? Why, of all the Spanish dances should the bolero be singled out to form the basis of the Spanish classical school? Perhaps it was because it was such a fine all-round dance, containing in addition to figures an endless variety of steps, at a time when the tendency in many countries at that time—England for example—was for dancers to be content with figures, steps being conspicuous by their absence.

The rise to favour may have been helped by the mania for arguing, criticizing and reading about dancing which was then fashionable. For eighteenth-century Spaniards, this was a new kind of diversion, and it is made clear in the literature of that time that they mistrusted the new 'ologies'. They were sceptical about 'method' when applied to their national dancing, for they were quite as convinced then as they are nowadays that Spanish dancing comes from the heart and not the head. Only towards the end of the century did they become dévotés of this 'school' which represented a different sort of discipline from that to which they were accustomed. Un-Spanish though it was, as an approach to dancing, it finally took root and, because it was not a Spanish concept, it could be written about with impunity; it might even, up to a point, be ridiculed as a dance form, especially when indulged in by foreigners.

Books on all kinds of dancing began to appear in greater numbers than before. Most of them dealt with social dancing and were directly inspired by French authors whom the Spaniards imitated. This spate of dance literature seems to imply that the Spanish people were taking a keen interest in examining and comparing their dances, and manner of dancing them, with other countries. This trend gave the moralists the opportunity they had always enjoyed, of continuing the age-old attack on dancing. They gleefully pointed out how perverse this new type of dancing could be, how it lacked decorum and, by stressing the lack of moral purpose, observed how Spanish standards would deteriorate if people persisted in falling victim to this alien diversion!

To sum up: with all this foreign 'danceology' in the air, the Spaniards could not avoid being affected by it. They were no longer content to merely dance; they thought, talked and wrote about varying standards and distinct values, as applied to dancing. This in the eighteenth century served the same purpose that 'public relations' does today. While discovering and at the same time disapproving of foreign systems of 'danceology', which more often than not, the Spanish intellectuals treated with scornful derision, they could not ignore them.

No dancing could excel Spanish dancing for vitality, nor the French style for elegance (pl. 28). Brought into contact with each other, a process of refinement was to be observed, first in the realm of Spanish social dance, which later extended to the Spanish theatre. When ballet as a developed art form was brought to Spain from abroad, it was produced with outstanding success. Magnificent repertoires were built up comparable, indeed in many ways similar, to those performed in opera houses abroad at the same period. With the ballets came foreign standards of production and criticism, but in them the hard kernel of Spanish dance always remained intact.

The new 'danceological' concepts did not affect the inherent beauty of Spanish dancing. Dancing was an emotional outlet for the Spaniards who loved and believed in their own dances with the same love and faith that they had for their country. Their main difficulty was to accept an intellectual approach to them. The mistrust of French intervention in the ballroom and, incidentally, intrusion into their social life, led to a renewal of their interest in the bolero. The presence of these dual influences at one and the same time, gave to the Spaniards a keener insight into dancing as a whole than they had possessed hitherto. Their outlook was still more broadened when the Italians took over the Spanish theatre and demonstrated practical means of adding valuable components to an already rich Spanish dance tradition. New methods of presentation improved the standard of Spanish stage dancing and the credit for rendering similar service to the cause of theatrical dancing, as the French had to ballroom dancing at the same period, must go to the Italians, as we shall see in the chapter that follows.

The dissemination of dance literature created a larger informed audience, ready, able, and eager to enjoy the ballets of alien extraction that later were to be so admirably adapted to Spanish taste in the Peninsula. The eighteenth century mania for 'ologies' in dancing turned out to be only a period of transition and, moreover, a most fruitful era for Spanish dancing as a whole.

6

Theatrical Dancing in Spain

WE HAVE already observed how, ever since the fifteenth century, the habit of adapting folk, ritual and court dancing to theatrical requirements had been slowly gaining ground. The presence of the French in eighteenth-century Spain exerted considerable influence upon Spanish dancing generally and undoubtedly speeded up the process of amalgamating the social and theatrical forms of dance. Spanish dancing might easily have continued to develop gently along these lines had not the Italians been brought to Spain to direct theatrical operations there.

Philip V was French, but his first two wives were Italian, and Italian influence soon became noticeable, even extending far beyond the confines of court life into the theatre. Italian dance masters were appointed to supervise ballet production. Not only that, they virtually dominated the theatres until the end of the century, adding fresh elements to those already existing—as might be expected from people with such long stage experience behind them.

The Italians knew well how to reconcile the regional style of dancing with their own correct academic discipline that was known as the 'Italian School'. Absorbing Spanish dances as fast as they could, they grafted their own theatrical concepts on the ancient tree of Spanish dance tradition and out of this grew the method of teaching which became world famous as the 'Spanish Classical Bolero School'. On this sound foundation, they were able to elaborate further the danced divertissements of the previous century and, eventually, succeeded in producing ballets consisting of three, four, or even five acts. Foot technique continued to develop and a system of arm movements came into being—both most useful adjuncts to the noble style of professional ballet dancing then fashionable in court theatres everywhere. The *grands ballets d'action* provided a perfect setting for them.

All these happenings came at a most opportune moment, for, early in the eighteenth century, more new theatres were being constructed all over Spain. This meant that Ballets could be presented under more favourable conditions than formerly. Permanent companies were attached to the theatres and were engaged to give regular performances. Most of these kept a dance group to provide the dances which were more often than not nothing more than incidental interludes in the operas, plays and comedies which were then so popular. As time went by, these dance groups became increasingly important, and dancing masters were contracted for the sole purpose of arranging dances. It was quite usual to find that special music was composed for the danced interludes or divertissements and, with a larger stage, the choreography developed accordingly.

Towards the middle of the century, real ballets were produced and, powerfully influenced by the Italians, became very grand and majestic. They were intended to be performed before audiences drawn from the upper ranks of society, headed, naturally, by the royal family. A sharp line divided the upper from the lower classes in Spain at that time, and the fact that the Italian artists were protected by their patronage guaranteed the acceptance of their art by court and aristocratic circles.

Opera and ballet thus flourished until the end of the century, by which time productions had become so ambitious, opulent and above all so expensive, that it was found quite impossible to subsidize them any longer. The theatre in Madrid specializing in these lavish spectacles closed, the company was disbanded and foreign artists were banned. Having made such a brilliant start and developed rapidly, this type of theatrical dancing later declined. A result of this slowing down of balletic progress was a come-back in favour of dancing of a popular, national kind which in time completely replaced the classical style in the theatre. As in the sixteenth century, whenever interludes were required, Spanish dancing was now demanded. Out of this change, another type of entertainment emerged, of modest dimensions and very Spanish in flavour. Known as a 'zarzuela' it was akin to what we might call an operetta today. The public loved it and finally adopted it in place of opera and ballet. There was plenty of dancing, as well as acting and singing, in this light form of entertainment and so it was, that the eighteenth century saw the rise of ballet as an art form and eventually, also, its decline.

To trace the movement in favour of theatrical dancing generally and, later, that of ballet in particular, let us return to the beginning of the century, when Philip V was on the throne. In 1703 and by royal command, an Italian company was engaged to perform at the Buen Retiro Theatre. Thereafter, Italian companies became a permanent feature of Spanish theatrical life. They alternated their performances with those given by Spanish companies. An influx of Italian musicians, actors, dancers, singers and scenic artists descended upon the Peninsula bringing with them their own plays and operas. At that time no Italian comedy was complete without some dances. The operas then fashionable also included danced divertissements, which finally were developed into full-length ballets.

A popular character in Italian comedy was Trufaldine and the first Italian company to settle in Madrid styled themselves Los Trufaldines, after him. The direction was granted permission to build on the site of the old wash-houses of Los Caños del Peral. There, they erected a wooden structure called the Corral de los Trufaldines which they opened in 1709, and in this way acquired their own theatre. Since they were under the king's protection, they paid no rent or taxes, a privilege that caused more than a little discontent among the Spaniards! Mutterings rose into a public outcry which soon led to a national protest against foreign artists, ending with the expulsion of the Italians from the country. Italian works, however, remained in fashion but they now had to be performed in Spanish. It is worth remarking that all the members of the dance group were Italian and, despite the ban, they stayed on.

The Corral de los Trufaldines then went through hard times; closing, opening, closing, only to reopen again. At last the theatre became the property of Madrid Town Council who restored, renovated and improved it. Inaugurated with a flourish in 1777, renamed the Corral de los Caños del Peral, it became a welcome addition to the other two corrales already in existence—the Principe and the Cruz. It also became the cradle of opera and ballet in Madrid and a resident company of musicians, dancers and singers performed there regularly. At first, the company was small, the dance group had only five women and six men, and the orchestra consisted of one leading violin, a second leading violin, and eight others. Two violas, two oboes, two horns and the basses completed the ensemble.

The season ran from 1 October, lasting until 1 July. Performances began at 7.30 p.m. and ended before 11 p.m. The theatre was administered with an efficiency that could scarcely be surpassed even in the present day—that is, if all the regulations set down on paper were carried out. These applied not only to the 'inside of the house', but extended to the behaviour of the audience outside the theatre; much thought had gone into a means of devising a satisfactory manner of controlling the traffic.

As far as the artists were concerned, encores were banned and the public could clamour for one in vain. No matter how distinguished the patrons were, they had to conform to this ruling. This must have cost the artists more than a little effort and self-restraint in those days of the 'star system'—indeed, to some, it must have been a positive test of endurance to contain themselves and comply!

In those days of wooden structures, strict precautions against fire had to be taken. Scenery was not permitted to be made of any inflammable material. In case of an outbreak of fire, pumps and vessels containing an adequate supply of water had to be ready and easily available. The Hospitals Commission was held responsible for their installation and maintenance. Why had the hospitals to concern themselves with this matter? Simply because they played an important part in the governing body of the municipal theatres in those days.

As for the audience in the front of the house, they had to conform to certain rules of conduct that the present day theatre-goer might find irksome, to say the least. Patrons in the stalls were strictly forbidden to chat or even signal to the ladies occupying the cazuela. Hats were not *de rigueur* and might not be worn either during the performances or the intervals. No smoking was allowed, a lighted cigar could not even be carried inside the theatre—a custom which still prevails in most opera houses. Ladies were charged to behave at all times with the decorous deportment fitting to their sex!

It was still customary for the ladies to sit in splendid isolation in the cazuela and there no gentleman ever set foot. This occupied half the theatre and it was enclosed by a balustrade. The tertulia occupied the other half and was destined for the men; needless to say, no women were allowed to enter there. Patrons of both the cazuela and the tertulia were requested to remain in their seats throughout the performance, unless they intended to leave the theatre for good; in which case, seats had to be vacated as quietly as possible during the interval. It would be difficult today to imagine any Spanish audience sitting through a whole performance without moving or changing places or flirting with the ladies and, a very tall order indeed, leaving quietly.

Anyone found guilty of misbehaving or falling below the standard of good manners then prevailing was liable to instant expulsion. Nobody could escape this ruling for it was by order of the mayor and no exception was made, even in the case of persons in the most exalted positions.

Outside the theatre, care was taken to see that traffic regulations were observed. To avoid all argument and prevent coachmen from jumping the queue, a picket of dragoons was posted nearby—by order of the military governor. Carriages had to wait in file along the streets adjoining the theatre but were not permitted to obstruct the square in which it was situated. Only very privileged people were allowed to park their vehicles there—patrons who might be hastily called away on urgent business as, for instance, the mayor or the superior of the Hospitals Commission.

It was the governing body of the hospitals that took charge of the administration—financial, artistic and, hardly necessary to add, moral. They allotted only two free boxes; one went to the court, the other to the mayor. Everybody else had to pay and boxes were allotted to important personalities according to their civic rank.

This was another ruling that applied to all, including the governor of the city, the magistrates and the superior of the hospitals.

At that time, the hospitals were staffed by members of religious orders and, since they were members of the governing body directing the municipal theatres, they were probably responsible for the stringent rules laid down concerning the behaviour of artists and audience and the well-ordered traffic arrangements. Nothing was left to chance. They kept a sharp eye on all performances to make quite sure that they maintained the high tone they demanded. A select committee of two, headed by the superior himself, inspected all productions and made it their business to insist that they conformed to current standards of 'decency'. Anything not measuring up to the canons of behaviour then prevailing, was banned at once. Any breach of good manners was condemned. If, by any chance, and in spite of the Vigilance Committee, something offensive appeared in any production, it was immediately reported to the mayor who had the power to prohibit any further public performance.

Once more we meet with this traditional censorship, and theatrical dancing then was just as liable to be prohibited as social dancing had been in the past, when any public exhibition of dancing was involved and tended to be regarded as suspect.

There was a certain note of dictatorship about the Hospitals Commission for they reserved the right to present dramatic plays on the days that opera was not being performed. In order to preserve Spanish art, they possessed full authority to substitute a Spanish work for an Italian and so benefit the national theatre. Italian opera predominated, but at no time was it permitted completely to monopolize the Spanish stage.

As far as the actual dance groups were concerned, it is clear that they were carefully organized and directed. Operatic works including elaborate dance divertissements demanded concentrated effort on the part of the management and this applied not only to the theatre in the capital, but elsewhere in Spain. Indeed, the constant changes that went on in the direction of various companies are quite bewildering to a modern reader. In 1752, the Hospital de Santa Cruz in Barcelona replaced the dance director and it is recorded that the group, consisting entirely of girls—although directed by a man—underwent many changes. The man was called 'El Monero', and in the same year he was replaced by one José Rubbini, who brought his relatives with him: Antonio, Andrés, Juan Batista Rubbini and Bartélemé Bartini. More changes were reported in this group also, possibly through too much family intervention. *Antigone* produced in 1753 was danced by three girls and three boys. The Rubbini family appeared in all the danced interludes performed in the numerous works produced in Barcelona.

The Catalans had the opportunity of hearing world-famous works by Porpora, Scarlatti and the other leading composers of the day. They prided themselves on this, and also that they heard and saw the great foreign artists long before they appeared in the capital and the rest of Spain. Opera flourished there, complete with the appended ballets, until the untimely deaths, first of the king and then the queen, put an end to the performances from 1759–60.

With the accession of Carlos III, another company was formed in Barcelona and this included a dance group directed by Gaudencio Beri. It consisted of four boys and four girls. The following year José Belluzi replaced Beri. *La Muchacha* was mounted in 1761 and later, the *Return from London*. Yet another director was appointed in 1762. The task of a dance director here appears to have been singularly arduous for not one of them stayed very long! In the same year, *La Astrologa* was produced and it was recorded that there were more comings and goings among the dancers. An interesting point indeed, for one characteristic of modern Spanish companies is that the dancers never stay in any one company long enough to become bored.

The new director was Italian. Four more Italian dancers were engaged and a choreographer named Inocencio Trabatteri arranged a 'heroic' and a 'comic' dance for the production of *Caton en Utica*. By 1767, nearly all the dancers were newcomers to the company and Francisco Guardini was appointed to direct the group. The Guardinis, husband and wife, presented a bullfight in dance form in *La Muchacha Lunatica*. The credit on the programme ran: 'Francisco and Teresa Guardini, virtuosi in the service of the Duke of Modena'. A supreme effort was made in 1769 to form a really impressive company, worthy of Barcelona. Directed by Felipe Chiari, an almost entirely new Italian group was engaged, and in the same year he arranged *La Noche Crítica* for nine dancers. In 1772, an augmented company was directed by Domingo Rossi, who was destined later to become so famous for his large, expensive companies in Madrid. Gluck's *Orfeo* was produced in 1780 but not until 1783, however, did an all-Spanish opera company emerge.

The invasion of the Spanish theatres by Italian artists and technical advisers of diverse kinds was by no means a temporary expedient, nor was it confined to the leading theatres in Madrid and Barcelona. This type of production, new to Spain and so peculiarly Italian, called for artists specializing in the interpretation of music and dancing in a certain manner, distinct from that formerly seen. In the hands of the Italians, stage dancing in Spain therefore underwent many changes and, in the process, developed still further.

Italian choreographers then, were very fond of what we today call 'demi-character' dancing; that is to say, a combination of mime and dancing. After the elegant and somewhat limited posturing, typical of theatrical dancing in the previous century, this freer form of movement somewhat altered the Spaniards' preconceived notions of dancing. In the past, there had been mimed branles and mime existed, but as a separate thing—an adjunct to dancing. Mime was considered sufficiently important in itself to necessitate engaging a special mime artist to perform, usually while the dancers had a rest. After 1750, things changed, for not only had dancers to dance, they had to be able to act and to express their emotion through mime as well as dancing. That required additional preparation and some extra training. The ballets continued to be divided into two basic categories; serious danced drama and comic ballet pantomime. Dancers were expected to be able to dance both comic and dramatic roles now, making added demands upon their powers of adaptation and versatility. Production as a whole was much more specialized; the Italians composed special music for the ballets, and lavish décor and costumes, with superb stage effects, were added. This all helped the dancers to portray more vividly than formerly their stories in movement, and a much more complete form of entertainment was gradually developed.

At that period, this type of production was receiving sustained ovations in various strongholds of ballet as, for example, in Paris, Vienna, Stuttgart and Milan. It did not take long for it to become equally successful in Spain, not only in the capital, but penetrating wherever a suitable theatre could be found in towns, both large and small.

In Cadiz, Alexander O'Reilly, who was the military governor, ordered a theatre to be built, the cost to be borne by wealthy citizens of the town, who in return were privileged permanently to control the allocation of the boxes. In 1761, a Venetian, Antonio Ribalba, directed the company and nearly all the dancers came from Milan. In the following year, he arranged the dances for *Andromaca*. Another Italian from Milan, Giuseppe Destefani, arranged the dances for *El Señor Doctor* in 1764. Two more changes were made in 1767, first when Juan Pablo Tomava was appointed dance director and, later, when Vicente Trabatere succeeded him. In 1769 Francisco Ferriano produced the ballet *El Bolognese* and ten dancers took part in this. Francisco Radetti arranged the dances in 1771. By 1792 the light opera company of Cadiz included not only a director but also the celebrated dancer and choreographer of those days, Agosto Favier. In the company were a ballerina *assoluta*, two leading soloists, who were *grotescos assolutos*, two other soloists of unspecified type and, to complete the group, there was a violin to accompany the dances. *The Italian in London* with music by Cimarosa was produced in 1792.

In eastern Spain, Valencia had two centres of theatrical activity: the Corral de Vall Hubert and the Corral Olivera. Unfortunately, the bishop was rather intolerant and so these corrales were demolished in 1761 after which date most operatic performances took place in the private theatre at the duke of Gandia's palace. In 1767, *L'Esclava Reconocida* with music by Piccini and dances by Belluzzi was produced. The dance group in 1769 was directed by Antonio Jansente and all six dancers bore Italian names. By 1774 Francisco Guardini, already mentioned with his wife dancing in Barcelona, turns up again as dance director, but we hear nothing more about his wife.

Even Mallorca boasted a dance group of its own; the director was Domenico Belliz, native of Bologna, and all the dancers hailed from Italy. In that home of dancing, Seville, the bishop forbade the performances of all comedies between 1779–90, but, curiously enough, he tolerated opera. Before the ban came into operation, Antonio Ribalta turned up in Seville in 1764 with a group of seven dancers and he was the choreographer.

In the north of Spain, a company appeared at Logroño headed by Juan Batista de Selveri, 'dance virtuoso in the service of His Excellency the Marquis of Montera'. He was the dance director of the Logroño company in 1764.

The foregoing list gives a fairly good impression of the widespread interest in theatrical dancing in various parts of Spain. The Italians appeared to play the leading role in propagating this art-form. Let us consider for a moment the underlying reason for this omnipresent influence in Spain that endured for so long, and then observe what Italian theatrical dancing consisted of at that time.

Why should the Spaniards be so attracted to Italian art? Why should Italian influence in this particular branch of theatrical art last such a long time? Quite apart from the fact that the royal houses of Spain and Italy had been united by marriage since the dawn of the eighteenth century, there was another reason why the taste for Italian art continued long after mid-century.

The first task of Carlos III, when he came to the throne in 1759, was to surround himself with good ministers who set to work to reorganize the administration of the country. The king had ruled the kingdom of Sicily since 1734 and it was perfectly clear that he fostered an appreciation for Italian art. Naples was then the capital—at a time, be it noted, when it was also the home of celebrated dancing masters. Not only had Carlos III learned to govern in Italy, he and his entourage had developed a taste for Italian art, with which they were perfectly familiar. It was during this reign, that lasted until 1788, that strong currents of Italian influence were seen to flow through the artistic and literary life of Spain.

The king personally was known for his love of hunting rather than dancing. Nevertheless, his reign turned out to be one of the most productive periods in the history of Spanish theatrical dance history. Stage dancing was passing through a period of transition everywhere in Europe just then. There was a general urge to liberate dancing from the constrictive formality of seventeenth-century concepts. Teachers were beginning actually to encourage their pupils to take longer steps, in opposition to the style obtaining in Pécour's day, when it was thought highly reprehensible to do so.[1] In the theatre, dancers now had to learn to cover the ground of the larger stages then under construction. To do this, they were forced to spread their movements. Flying steps were typical of the bolero, so they suited this purpose admirably and the Italians were quick to realize their value.

Some useful information about the way in which the changes from the old fashioned conception of stage dancing were realized, is to be found in the Italian *Trattate prattico di balle* by the cele-brated maestro Magri published in 1788. Here, the stilted move-ments typical of the early eighteenth-century technique are com-pared with the 'modern manner' of dancing. Broadening the movements was one characteristic; another, was a different way of 'timing' the steps. When airing his views on the cruel limitations imposed upon dancing in the old days, the maestro refers to himself as one of 'we moderns'. A startling innovation—or so it seems today, when we use only five positions of the feet—were the ones he listed; no fewer than twenty-five are described!

Among others, we discover five 'Spanish positions' in which the feet are neither turned out or in, but are kept in a straight line. The five 'true' or turned-out classical positions are noted and also, the five 'false' or turned-in positions. The five 'forced' positions are interesting in that they are not of any determined length; that is to say, the length of one's own foot—as in the past. The five positions 'in the air' speak for themselves.

This insistence on the various angles of the feet indicates that the maestro was much concerned with the study of 'line' since these diverse angles of the dancers' feet fundamentally affected the positions, thereby completely altering the dancers' movements. All these changes concerning the line, direction and timing of steps were leading to a freer conception of movement as a whole than

---

[1]Pécour made his début at the Paris Opera House in 1672. Later, he became famous as dancing master.

had been possible formerly. It is significant that this trend was in line with the general leaning, then prevalent, towards greater freedom of thought in other human activities. No longer confined to Feuillet's limited notation, new steps came into existence, many of them being of Spanish origin. Dancers had a wider choice as, one by one, the shackles of early eighteenth-century dances were shed. It seems obvious that the addition of Spanish steps to those of the old Italian academic repertoire contributed much to the progress of stage dancing. The Italians, taking the trouble to describe and specially note the five Spanish positions, and adding them to their own, proves how seriously they regarded Spanish dancing and their interest in it. In adopting Spanish positions they enlarged the scope of their own work. Whilst in Spain, they moulded their ideas to suit Spanish taste and the Spaniards returned the compliment, by endeavouring to master the Italian conception of foot technique.

The interchange of ideas with the rest of Europe, obvious in the sphere of social dancing in the eighteenth century, now extended to that of the theatre; an important development just then, when a vogue for classical ballet was spreading through European theatres, especially those attached to the larger royal courts. Through her dance tradition Spain made a vast contribution to the type of choreography then being utilized in those productions. It was quite usual to find entire themes for ballets centred on Spain, or based on Spanish legends and heroes. Spanish influence in the domain of dance instruction, also, is clearly demonstrated in the textbooks written by Italian dancing masters, who described the Spanish manner of dancing and apparently considered it quite as important as the French and Italian styles.

As for the Spanish people, they did not always receive this exchange of ideas with enthusiasm. Court circles patronized the ballet with delight, a delight not shared by the Spanish artists employed in the theatres! In the first place, this was because the boleros and boleras were poorly paid by comparison with the foreigners, who, not content with this, cornered the leading roles and also brought their families with them—to monopolize the key positions in the companies! Entire families are still employed nowadays in Spanish groups and this is generally regarded as a gypsy custom, but it might well be a remnant of Italian tradition which, like Italian technique, lingers on.

Painful as it was to the artists, many members of the general public also found this process of integration equally objectionable chiefly for patriotic reasons. It took some time to convince a Spaniard of conventional taste, versed in his own dancing, that this alien style of dancing was any better than his own, and still more difficult to convince him that anything could replace the familiar old jotas, fandangos and seguidillas. That this developed form was fashionable in France or Italy was not sufficient recommendation in itself; Spaniards felt it was unpatriotic to encourage foreign entertainment. At first the only section of the community to whom ballet really appealed was the sophisticated well-travelled set, who enjoyed it primarily because it was non-Spanish—being foreign made it all the more attractive to them. Only in the last quarter of the century did people from all walks of life begin to accustom themselves to watch ballets and then they were captivated by the magic and ultimately fell under the spell of their irresistible beauty. National prejudice had by then been overcome, and theatre-going Spaniards were transformed into regular balletomanes. Once accepted by the general public, this strange, unfamiliar entertainment prospered, becoming ever more grandiose and this is what led to its ultimate downfall.

The great protagonist in the realm of spectacular ballet production in Spain was a former pupil of Noverre's. He was the Italian dancer Domingo Rossi, and was engaged as dancer, choreographer and ballet master at the Teatro de los Caños del Peral in Madrid. At one point, he was in charge of the opera as well and, as he was in a position of dictator, it was not long before ballet became all-important and the opera purely incidental! As his ballets became more spectacular more money was needed, for Rossi's *corps de ballet* was famous for its size—far too large for a small town like eighteenth-century Madrid, so his critics claimed. Nevertheless, even though he nearly ruined them in the process, this was the man who revealed to the Spaniards what ballet in the grand manner really was. His repertory closely followed Noverre's whose ballets were then so successful in France, Italy and Austria and perhaps this is why he accomplished his task so brilliantly. In addition to his official appointment, he ran a private training school of his own and did not hesitate to use his pupils from this establishment to augment the Opera Ballet. This caused endless dissatisfaction, especially at one point, when there were only seven artists in the opera, with a chorus of twelve, while a huge *corps de ballet* was padded with various members from the 'director's school'.

The themes of Rossi's *ballets d'action* followed the current fashion of the time and were either of a tragic, comic or heroic nature. On 9 December 1788, he produced the *Judgment of Paris* in honour of Her Royal Highness the Princess of Asturias. An enormous caste was involved in this production, and in addition to many principal dancers were retinues of heroes attending the gods and goddesses, shepherds and shepherdesses, zephyrs, genies, pleasures, as well as trains of various abstract figures of an earthly, celestial, maritime and infernal nature. The ballet told the story of Paris and the golden apple and was in three acts. It ended with a magnificent apotheosis scene, when golden clouds descended from above and a portrait of the princess could be discerned among the sunbeams. Venus at once indicated that the apple belonged to one person and laid it at the foot of the royal portrait, then retinues of goddesses garlanded it around with flowers. A general dance concluded the scene, to commemorate the glorious day of the Princess of Asturias —'our beloved lady, long may she live'.[2]

The season opened the following year with *Los Varones de Rocca*; *A Village Wedding*, and a grand divertissement in which the entire company danced. Juan and Maria Medina, two dancers from Madrid who later were to become famous, danced for the first time, and Rossi made many changes by rearranging existing dances in the repertoire: he took some from *Don Quixote and Sancho Panza* to arrange for *Las Bodas de Sancho*, produced others for *Los Dos Condes* with music by Cimarosa, and inserted one comic and one heroic dance in *Semiramis*.

[2]An original copy of this libretto exists in the library of the royal palace, Madrid. By kind permission of the Patrimonio Nacional I was permitted to consult and quote from it.

A prolific choreographer, he did not confine himself only to allegorical themes; following the general European trend, he utilized rustic themes as well as those that dealt with the lives of ordinary mortals. They were such an excellent pretext for arranging suites of popular national and character dances. The following list gives some idea of his range: *La Fiesta Tirolesa, Feria Napolitana, Baile Inglés, Faxal de Renfrew, La Esposa Persiana, Las Diversiones Campestres, Máscaras de Bologna, Los Provenzales, El Prado de Madrid, Los Gitanos Sorprendidos, Cleopatra, Campamiento de los Hungaros, Fiesta Persiana, Recreaciónes Polacas* and *La Fille Malgardée*.

Like many other ballet masters before and since his time Rossi appears to have had some difficulty in imposing discipline upon his dancers! The following letter from Teresa Mazzonetti-Montesini implies that he was too nervous to deliver his message to her in person, since the order was conveyed to her by her husband. She answered: 'My husband tells me that you request me to modify my wearing apparel in the ballet that is being given tonight. I am prepared to meet your demand with one exception, and that is that I will not alter the type of ballet slippers I wear. I can only dance with complete freedom in knitted slippers [malle] and I will not do as you suggest and change to satin ones. I am quite prepared to dance in my own knitted slippers but absolutely refuse to appear in silk ones. I am notifying you of this in good time. My husband made a special concession in wearing them for the Capuchetty benefit performance and nothing less would have induced him to do so.'

As foot technique became more involved it was found necessary to reinforce ballet slippers to give some support to the feet; this was achieved in the first place by stiffening the shoes and making them from firmer material. Rossi appears to have been making some effort to bring the dancers in Spain into line with the rest of Europe in this matter. Soft woven slippers were gradually giving way to stiffer satin or canvas pumps for stage wear and these were sometimes reinforced by darning. The greater the technical demands made upon the dancers, the more necessary this support became, and it was this tendency that in time led to blocking the shoes as dancers rose higher and higher on the ball of the foot until they were actually dancing on tip-toe. These satin slippers were really the forerunners of the blocked ballet shoes that arrived in the nineteenth century. A sigh of sympathy can almost be heard from ballet students through the ages for the eighteenth-century ballerina who defied authority in staking her claim for comfortable feet when dancing.

Rossi's troubles were not confined to footwear alone. Dress regulations in Spain then were strict and presented a problem. The authorities were still very concerned about what was and what was not 'decent'. The Spaniards were not yet quite ready to accept the kind of innovation La Camargo made about 1730, when she shortened her skirt to cut the first entrechat which set a fashion that nearly everybody in the dancing world hastened to copy in the leading European theatres. Not so in Spain, however, for the managements would not even permit flesh coloured tights to be worn, unless the dancers covered them up with long skirts! They were quite determined that audiences should be given no cause for offence. They decreed that in the theatre 'decency' might not be sacrificed upon the altar of technical prowess. Spanish dancers just had to put up with the encumbrance of weighty skirts and do the best they could.

Rossi had plenty of criticism lavished upon him which does not appear to have perturbed him unduly, since he did nothing to combat it. As might be expected, the growing taste for opera and ballet brought critics as well as admirers to the fore. The reputation of a dancer could be built up in print and destroyed with equal facility! Dance critics in those days were somewhat more verbose than they are nowadays. They did not hesitate to hurl invective, carry on lively arguments with violent explosions of rhetoric, or play on the heartstrings of their readers by appealing to their emotions.

Two celebrated dancers of the day were involved in one exuberant outburst. They were La Medina, the Spanish dancer (and wife of Salvador Vigano who was Boccherini's nephew) and the Italian dancer La Pelosini. Pelosini had disappointed one section of the Press who claimed that she no longer fulfilled the promise she had

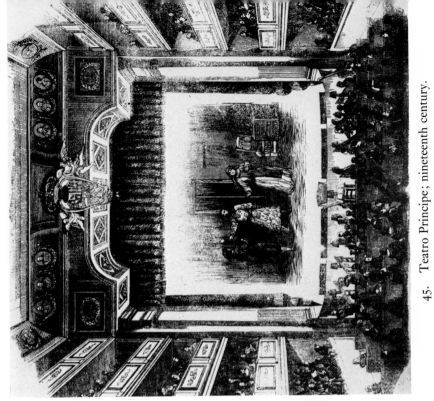

45.   Teatro Principe; nineteenth century.

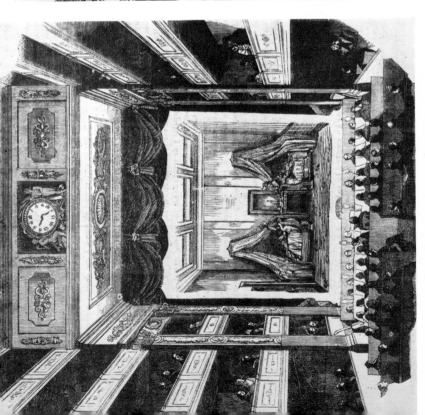

44.   Teatro de la Cruz; nineteenth century.

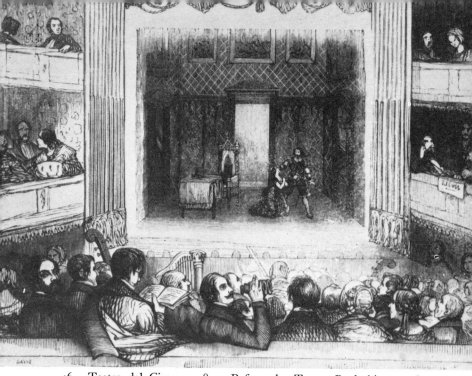

46. Teatro del Circo *c.* 1842. Before the Teatro Real this was the most important theatre for operatic productions in Madrid. Marie–Guy Stephan was partnered by Petipa here.

47. Romantic ballet in nineteenth century Spain. Pas de Jrois.

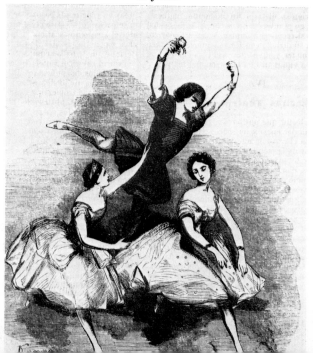

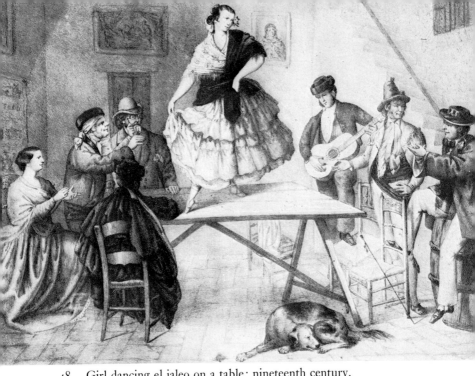

48.   Girl dancing el jaleo on a table; nineteenth century.

49.   *Baile del candil* danced indoors; late eighteenth century.

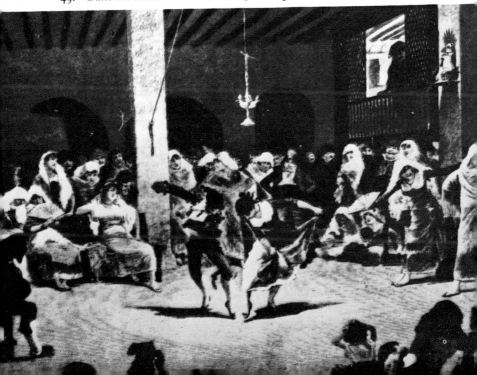

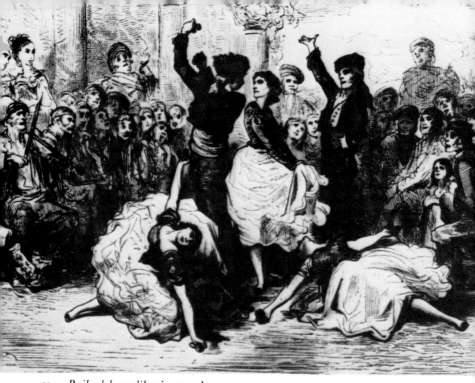

50. *Baile del candil*; nineteenth century.

51. Couple dancing el gitano before a local audience; nineteenth century.

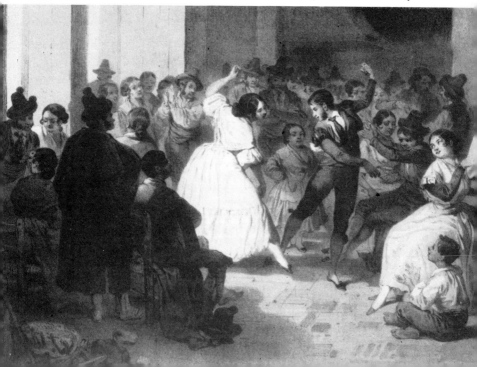

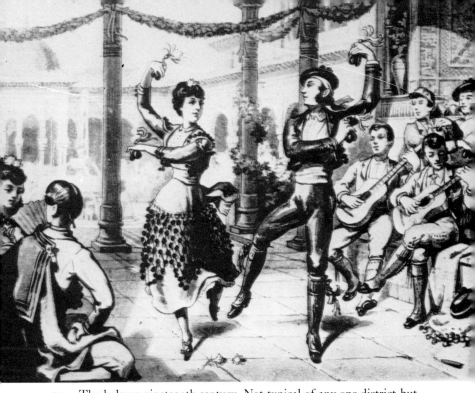

52. The bolero; nineteenth century. Not typical of any one district but containing everything characteristic of Spanish dancing.

53. Teatro Real, 1868.

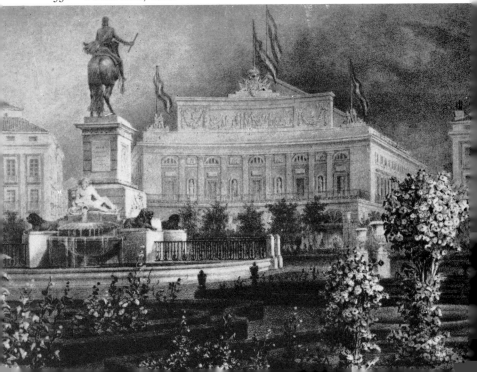

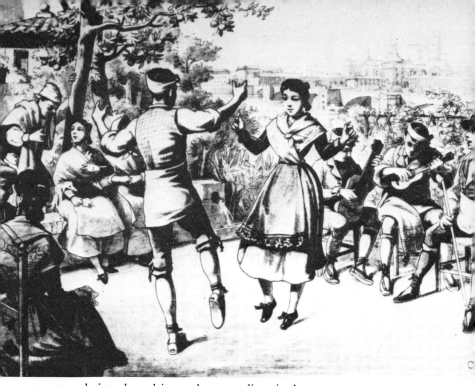

54. la jota danced in rural surroundings in Aragon.

55. Jota Navarra (El Chun-Chu). Note difference in carriage of arms in this Jota and that of Aragon (pl. 54).

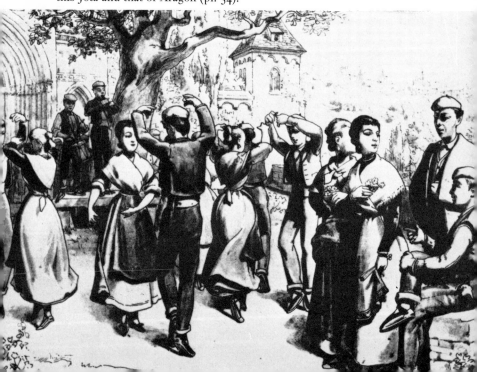

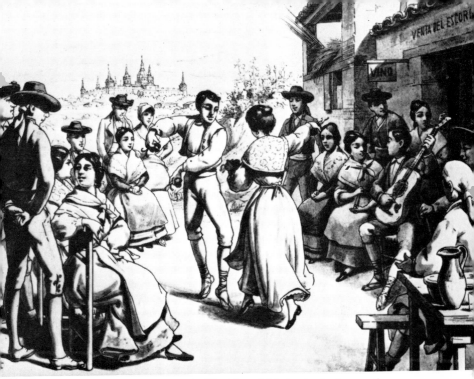

56. The seguidilla (New Castille). The Esconial is in the background.

57. El fandango (Audalucia), danced in native surroundings.

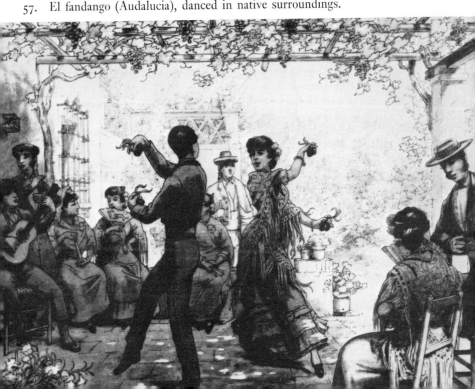

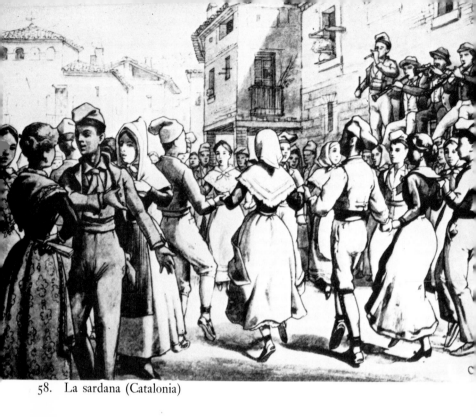

58. La sardana (Catalonia)

59. La danza prima (Asturias).

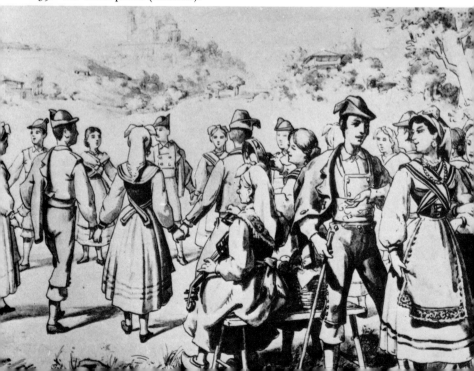

shown at the outset of her career. Not only this, they solemnly warned her that she would only draw applause from her audiences for as long as she could dance her fandango with castanet accompaniment. Further, they told her to avoid forcing herself to do the beats and cabrioles that her obesity (sic) prevented her from performing successfully. They even threatened her that if she persisted in trying to do these steps, she would be more than ever unfavourably compared with La Medina, whose transcending excellence lay in her beaten work. (Maria Medina's champions boasted that it was her technical strength allied to her natural grace and charm that justified the continuous applause that always greeted her.)

Pelosini's admirers were not going to suffer that sort of eulogy in silence and replied with vigour: 'Pelosini's mime is a prodigious expression of truth—her burning glances and gestures spoke to the enraptured audiences when she acted. Why! she is acclaimed now as she was at the commencement of her career; she dances now as she did then, she fills the theatres now as she always did. This was the 'Diario's' verdict and since it is correct, the public neither denies or contradicts it.'

This reference to the impression Pelosini's mime made upon her audience, serves to remind one of the importance this element played in the *grands ballets d'action* during the last quarter of the century. Mime in the past had been used in ballets as a separate entity, a purely incidental accessory. It was early in the eighteenth century that a change took place and the dancing masters, in their search for a means of liberating ballet from the old routine of entrances—noble and otherwise—with their suitable exits, following monotonous suites of dances, that had satisfied people for so long, hit upon the idea of combining mime with dancing, thereby discovering what a useful device this was to help them achieve their end. Then it was that facial expression, gesture, a more expressive use of the upper part of the body all became just as essential to dancers' technique for stage dancing, as was their neat, clean footwork. By the time that Noverre had revolutionized eighteenth-century ballet by introducing exaggerated mime and fusing it with pure dancing, a good deal of experimental work had already been carried out, for this problem had for some time preoccupied many of his predecessors.

The enormous success that greeted Noverre's productions about 1760, gave to the world and set a formula for classical ballet production that has remained in fashion ever since. But, in widening the range of the dancers' interpretation in this way, even he laid himself open to much criticism. In Spain, opinion was divided, for while some people admired the Noverian works, others yearned for pure dancing alone, when Spanish dancing was concerned, which most Spaniards agreed was complete in itself.

The eruption of the Pelosini-Medina dispute underlines the feeling of the two schools of thought on the subject; opinions were still divided. Of the Spanish Maria Medina one contemporary wrote: 'With her tender expressive movements and natural simple air, what a treasure of grace she is! Her ports de bras and sweet little turns of the head are admirable. Her sudden, significant little capers are enough to make even the steeliest heart palpitate. One could not discuss her without recalling those imponderably sublime beaten steps, wherein lay such grace and skill—surely the invention of art alone and juvenile mischief.'

Perhaps the most interesting feature of these dissertations is that the Italian dancer, Pelosini was criticized for her lack of technical skill, usually associated with Italian training, whereas her Spanish colleague, La Medina, was admired for her strong technique, which quite possibly was due in part to some help given her by her Italian husband, Vigano. Pelosini was praised by Spanish critics for accompanying her Spanish dances with the castanets; that she had gone to the trouble of mastering this intricate component of Spanish dancing no doubt flattered them.

Another interesting detail about these comments by the critics of the day is the allusion to the graceful way in which La Medina used the head and arms when she danced. They too were beginning to realize the importance of this part of dance technique. The French masters of that period in particular, were most insistent upon the correct use of arms, head and body when dancing. In the late seventeenth and early eighteenth centuries, they had been responsible, as we have seen, for introducing this facet of technique into the social dances of Spain. Dancers were already accustomed to co-ordinate their arms with footwork, and in the first quarter of the century an elaborate system of arm movements came into being, closely related to the positions of the feet which, by then, were clearly defined. These arm movements were the forerunners of the port de bras which every ballet student has to learn today.

In 1735, the French master Rameau described the carriage of the arms in his book *Le Maître à Danser* published in Paris. 'The arms should be as a frame to the body', he wrote. His system consisted of a basic position of the arms which was at the side of the body and to which position the arms must return between other movements. In Spanish dancing, this position has been retained exactly in the form he described, whereas in classical ballet it has become obsolete or, shall we say, modified, since the arms in the basic classical position, instead of being at the side of the body, are held over the thighs. The use of the head and shoulders known to ballet students as 'épaulement' is identical in Spanish dancing with that described in the eighteenth century—an important link with Rameau, for 'shading' as described by him, although still employed in classical ballet technique, is used sparingly. Another connection with French eighteenth-century academic technique, very prevalent in Spanish dancing, and almost obsolete in classical ballet today, is the circling of the wrists. This is very typical of Spanish dancing, so much so that most laymen associate this with 'flamenco arms'—or those movements commonly found in Spanish gypsy dancing.

The fact that, in Spanish dance technique, the carriage of the arms, head and shoulders, and their use when co-ordinated with the feet, corresponds so closely to those described by Rameau makes one suspect that he may have played a major role in influencing the development of Spanish ports de bras. He was certainly in a good position to do so, since he was in the service of Philip V's second Italian wife, Isabel of Farnese. It seems highly probable that Rameau's teachings profoundly affected Spanish court dancing in the early part of the eighteenth century and, subsequently, were incorporated into theatrical dancing by the Italians, as the process of adapting the dance material they found in Spain to the cause of their developed form of stage dancing evolved; a point well worth looking into.

During the time that the Italians were kept busy in the Spanish theatres, ever seeking new ways of fitting Spanish dancing into the framework of their stage requirements, dance influences from France were ever present. Style was all important at that period and it was considered smart to know the latest French variations. Paris remained supreme in the world of fashion and not only were the social dances that were imported from there eagerly copied, so was the French manner of dancing them—which we had reason to observe in the previous chapter. This was the case of social dances which, as formerly, continued to find their way into the theatre. Thus, it came about that in the eighteenth-century Spanish theatres dancing in the French, Italian and Spanish manner existed side by side. Maestro Magri, in his treatise, wrote of Vigano performing a 'cabriole à la française and ending it à l'espagnole and thereby creating a sensation'.

The shortening of the dancers' skirts took place in France about 1730 and most people seem to think that this did more than anything else to help along the development of classical ballet technique, with particular reference to foot technique. Progress in Spain in this direction must have been somewhat slower than elsewhere for, as we have seen, Spanish convention forbade their dancers wearing short skirts at that early date. Until the authorities controlling the theatres lifted the ban, the dancers could not be expected to perform more intricate technical feats and so this might account for the men having more opportunity to shine in this particular sphere, technical prowess among the ladies being left to the more emancipated foreign ballerinas. The freedom of movement that was gaining ground in other European countries came much later in Spain and only became characteristic of the famed Spanish Bolero School towards the end of the century (pl. 24).

On the interpretive side, the urge to express movement through conventional mime at the same time as dancing brought Spanish ballets into line with the style then contemporary in France and Italy. This, amalgamated with French arm movements, Italian foot technique, and traditional Spanish dance material produced a highly original, stylized form of dance composition. With its elaborated sequence of steps, intricate variations of movements and ground patterns, allied to the added adornment of castanet accompaniment, a 'modern' style was born that captured the imagination of dancers everywhere and subsequently penetrated the theatres of the world, outside Spain.

As may be imagined, the Italians, revelling in the vast quantity of indigenous dance material they found in Spain, set to work and produced a highly developed form of dance that found an outlet in their balletic productions that, as time went by, became grander and more flamboyant than ever. Too grand by far, when Rossi was in charge, or so the government felt, for his visions of grandeur nearly ruined them. They decided to put a stop to his extravagance.

At the Teatro de los Caños del Peral, Rossi produced two Noverre works in 1790: *Orpheus and Eurydice* and *Adèle de Fonthieu* set to music by Cimarosa. Rossi had already produced these ballets in Vienna and Milan (in 1770 and 1776 respectively). He retired from the Spanish theatre after reviving them, or rather he was obliged to relinquish his post and a singer was appointed to direct the opera in his place. A completely new company was formed and Agosto Favier was asked to run the ballet. He did—first by appointing himself and his wife as the first dancers *assolutos*. The company was completed by one other first dancer, two first soloists, two *grotescos*, three understudies and a *corps de ballet*. Despite this new appointment the joint opera and ballet company continued to lose money. It was hinted that, like Rossi, the new director was only interested in feathering his own nest. Losses to the hospitals continued.

Domingo Rossi returned to his old post in the following year, with new honours. Now known as 'Don Domingo', he added to his vast array of soloists, a *corps de ballet* of eighteen, sixteen extras and six boys from his own school. Combining acting, dancing and conventional mime in his own notoriously lavish manner, his new productions surpassed in magnificence anything he had ever done in the past. He set to work to utilize the entire range of mythology and continued to produce four- and five-act ballets which, needless to say, all involved ever increasing expenditure. Taking elaborate stories as themes, he allowed his imagination to run away with him. An instance of this was his *Iphigenía*, the ballet Noverre performed in London when he sought refuge in England after the French revolution. Others produced in the same extravagant vein were *L'Alzire*, *La Dama Soldada*—a tragi-comic ballet so we are told, presented on the occasion of Teresa Manzonetti's benefit performance, that famous girl who championed the 'comfortable slippers for dancers' campaign.

Rossi was in the habit of expounding his ballets at great length in Spanish-Italian prose. The libretti remain but no musical scores, which is a pity for these might have helped us to assess the length of the acts in these five-act epics which, by present day standards, appear rather long. Cimarosa appears to have been highly favoured as a composer for ballets; many of his scores exist in the Royal Palace Library, Madrid, but apparently there are no specially commissioned ballet scores available at present for reference. This does not mean that they may not exist, or be hidden away somewhere. The important thing to remember about these lengthy ballet productions, which appear to have been complete in themselves is, that in the following century, this was the theatre that became the Royal Opera House when it was rebuilt on the same site. The cradle of Spanish classical ballet was no other than the eighteenth-century Teatro de los Caños del Peral.

The continuous losses incurred sealed the fate of the theatre and, incidentally, as far as Spain was concerned, that of Rossi. The cost of mounting his increasingly ambitious ballet productions was too heavy. The government was not disposed to subsidize foreign artists indefinitely and so they finally decided to close the theatre. Rossi, representing as he did the extravagant era in which he lived and worked, was a visionary with unbounding enthusiasm which he seemed unable to control and he overreached himself. All the criticism levelled at him was concerned with the excessive expense of costumes, décor and a large company of dancers with a salary sheet reaching astronomical proportions for those days. It was further suggested that the director himself took the lion's share! His prodigality knew no bounds and the more successful his ballets, the more he proceeded to devise ever more costly scenic effects which, in turn, brought in their wake too many other incidental expenses. They reached such alarming dimensions that they had to be discontinued.

On 18 December 1799, an official decree disbanded the theatre on the grounds that it could not exist without substantial government support which was no longer forthcoming. So the theatre was closed. Later, a Spanish company replaced the Italian, but for some time it was minus a dance group. The following conditions were laid down for the future:

1 Any profits accruing from the lease of the theatre had to be donated to the hospitals.

2 Spanish works only had to be performed and in Spanish; any dancing therein to be from the 'Three Kingdoms'.

It was perfectly clear that henceforward, only *baile nacional* would be permitted and ballet in the classical sense fell into oblivion for the time being. The Spanish public, deprived of this expensive luxury, then turned their attention to the typically Spanish form of entertainment already alluded to, known as the 'zarzuela'.

The name 'zarzuela', came from the hunting lodge of that name, situated in the royal domain of El Pardo outside Madrid. This had been used by the royal family ever since the seventeenth century as a country retreat and there it was that zarzuelas were born. Originally, they were in the form of miniature masques with danced interludes in between the action of the play. The Italians had had a hand in their development in the previous century, but by the time the eighteenth century dawned, zarzuelas were being devised by Spaniards based on Spanish themes—in addition to the others of non-Spanish origin—and Spanish music was composed to accompany them. They came to be regarded as a typically Spanish art form. Being of modest dimensions, they were economical to produce and the national flavour appealed to the public who evinced the same affection for them as audiences in England do for ballad opera of the Gilbert and Sullivan type. Above all, zarzuelas were bright and cheerful and were popular enough to merit a special theatre to be devoted to their production being built in Madrid, called appropriately enough the Zarzuela.

Once again, Spanish dancing in the theatre was all the rage. To suit the taste of the new audiences it was modified into light danced divertissements, always bearing a distinctly national bias. Dance technique was not nearly so important as effective presentation.

Simple folk-dances were furbished with accessories of the shawl, cape, fan and flower variety. Fans and shawls were much sought after in the eighteenth century and as for capes—bullfighting and otherwise—they were almost a uniform. Business with the colonies was brisk at that period and shawls from Manila and fans from the Philippines invested the dances with an exotic whiff of distant lands. Added colour and movement was needed and no dance on the stage was complete without one or all of these accessories.

This in turn led to the dancers having to re-orientate their ideas and review their approach to stage dancing. Castanets were, as ever, the classical accompaniment to the dances, footwork was as important as ever, and in addition dancers now had to manipulate this added paraphernalia—which is not as easy to do as one might think. This was another angle on dancing for, unless skilfully handled, the accessories could deteriorate into being no more than an impediment to the dances, instead of an ornament. The dancers had to keep a steady rhythm with their feet, while doing something else with the upper part of the body—possibly in a totally different rhythm— and they were expected to keep an even flow of movement throughout the dance. This new facet of stage-craft demanded just as much attention as had the evolution of steps in the past, or the development of dance form (shape and figures in the ground patterns). Zarzuela audiences wanted variety, colour and movement in their stylized national dances and this is what the dancers gave them.

In retrospect, it seems strange that classical ballet production, after having reached such a high peak of development in eighteenth-century Spain, the traditional home of dancing, should fall into abeyance. Particularly since this coincided with a period of great balletic progress in the rest of Europe, where classical ballet continued to develop. It had taken a long time to evolve and the fine interplay of Spanish-French-Italian influences contributed much to the expansion of the seventeenth-century *ballets de cour* into the eighteenth-century *grands ballets d'action*. Yet, as we have seen, it took only a very short time to disappear. The long, ballet productions in Spain, at their best, were comparable to those produced in France and Italy, and the Spanish kind had the advantage of possessing their own school of Spanish dance technique, unique at the time but, due to an untimely theatrical end, never reaching complete maturity. The lack of an established theatre and a national ballet to keep it alive was responsible for this.

Throughout the centuries, a chain of dance tradition had been forged in Spain but a link with the theatre was broken in 1799, with the closing of the theatre and the dismissal of the Italians. The eighteenth century ended on a sad note from a balletic point of view and a glittering epoch in the annals of Spanish theatrical dancing was brought to a close when the Teatro de los Caños del Peral was demolished.

The arrival of the nineteenth century found Spain confronted once more with internal upheavals and the country was torn by the convulsions of war. There were matters far more grave to consider than the formation of a national ballet. People had neither thought, inclination nor money for this purpose. All was not yet lost, however, for, halfway through the century, at about the same time the Bolshoi Theatre was being reconstructed in Russia, a decision was made to build a new opera house in Madrid.

Built on the site formerly occupied by the Teatro de los Caños de Peral, the title of 'Real' or Royal Opera House was bestowed upon it. Apparently, what had at one point seemed to be a break with tradition turned out to be no more than a temporary deviation. Now that there was a large opera house in the capital, the Spaniards naturally hoped that the truly national theatre they had so earnestly desired for so long, would at last come into being. Yet, this was not to be, for it soon became clear that nothing had been learned from the mistakes of the past! Very soon, the Real was inundated by foreign artists of diverse kinds. Another public outcry ensued, louder than before and this time directed at the Government no less, for permitting such an anomaly. Evidently, a huge subsidy was allotted to finance the foreign stars of international fame which the snob audiences of that establishment demanded should appear, while at the same time, the Zarzuela Theatre, fighting to sponsor Spanish artists and talent, as well as exclusively presenting national works, received no official support whatsoever!

The Zarzuela Theatre functions nowadays, as it did in the old days. Zarzuelas continue to fill the theatre, whereas opera and ballet do not. There are more theatres in Madrid today than in any other big Spanish city but neither the opera nor the ballet seems to appeal to the Spanish theatre-going public. The fight for theatrical supremacy goes on continuously between the capital and Barcelona, and the latter town has the obvious advantage of being the proud possessor of a grand opera house with a large stage, which is frequented by visiting ballet companies.

It is well known that serious attempts were made to found a stable company after the establishment of the Royal Opera House in Madrid during the last century. This much we know, but the reason why neither opera nor ballet succeeded in taking root there, with any degree of permanency, has been overlooked. In the following chapter, some causes of the failure will be dealt with.

7

Spanish Dance Influence at Home and Abroad

EARLY IN the nineteenth century, the situation in Spain was such that any further development of Spanish ballet was out of the question. Occasionally, visiting companies from abroad gave short seasons of ballet, but life generally was too unsettled for the people to evince much interest in that kind of dancing.

Throughout the first half of the century, this state of affairs continued right up to the time that the Royal Opera House was opened in Madrid. The presence of the Real gave some sort of stability to the theatrical scene even though it proved to be of a temporary nature. It soon became apparent that, as in the previous century, the Real was to become a haven for foreign artists. Inevitably this again led to complaints, recrimination and general dissatisfaction. That this could be allowed to happen, after the experiences in the past, and in view of the unsettled state of the country, it seems extraordinary to us today that foreign artists were tolerated at all.

The fact that the Peninsula had been ravaged by the Napoleonic Wars and that the Spanish people were consumed with ardent nationalism before and immediately afterwards, did not appear to have the slightest effect in preventing companies from abroad working in Spain. As early as 1806, we find a French company in Madrid, dancing at the Principe Theatre (pl. 45)—now the Teatro Español. Vestris was with them during that season and the company presented *Danzomania* and *Gavotte*. In 1808 yet another French company appeared headed by François Lefèbre, presenting the well-known *Fille Malgardée*, *The Judgment of Paris*, *Folies d'Espagne* and *Don Quixote*.

About that time there was a movement on foot to try to hispanicize the Noverian ballets, and it was realized that some training would have to be provided for the dancers to be prepared for this specialized branch of theatrical art. In 1807, the extravagant Domingo Rossi was invited to form the instructional establishment. The idea was to limit it to sixteen girls and boys between the ages of eight and sixteen. History intervened, however, for in the following year Spain was again invaded and the whole scheme had to be abandoned. The Spaniards were to be kept far too busy for some time, defending their homeland first and later their colonies, to spare a thought for training schools!

It has been observed in the past that war is often followed by a period of dance mania, and Spain confirmed this observation. After Madrid had been liberated from French occupation, dancing became so immensely popular that from 1808 onwards there was a general recall to Spanish dancing among the ordinary people. Emotions were still running high and love of country was identified with love of Spanish songs and dances. Boleros, fandangos, jotas of every conceivable kind—and there were many variations—were danced with renewed zest and vigour, all over the country. The theatre once more showed new signs of life and *baile nacional* was the favourite form of dancing there.

At that time there was a popular performer called La Molina, famous alike for her dancing and her love affair with the Corregidor of Madrid. So many scandalous jokes began to circulate concerning the amorous adventures of these two, that the authorities finally put a stop to them by forbidding any reference to them in public, by law. This is of interest to dancers for the book of the *Three Cornered Hat* is said to have been based on this alleged liaison.

Anti-French feeling continued long after the occupying forces had been with drawn from Spain, yet the attitude of the people towards French dancing remained much the same as in the past. The Spaniards continued dancing the social dances from France that had become so popular in the Spanish ballrooms. As for the theatre, French companies paid regular visits (pls. 34, 47).

In 1818, Vestris returned with his group and mounted a one-act version of *Don Quixote* with eight variations and a ballet entitled *Mazourka* whose title was later changed to *Polka Mazourka*. The year 1818 was important in Spanish theatrical history for it was in that year that the foundations were laid in Madrid for the Royal Opera House. Unfortunately, building operations had to be suspended and finally ceased altogether in 1820! In 1830 the architect died. After that, the shell of the building was used for a variety of purposes ranging from a gunpowder store and a guards barracks to parliamentary sittings and masked balls! Thus it came about that, deprived of any hope of a permanent home in the capital, theatrical dancing once more fell to a low ebb. Such interest as there was, was barely kept alive by the rare visits of foreign companies. When the writer Théophile Gautier was visiting Spain in the late 1830s, he was amazed at the dearth of good dancing and this prompted him to observe: 'At Burgos, Vittoria and Valladolid we are told that the great dancers are in Madrid. In Madrid we are informed that they are in Andalucia or Seville; we shall see. I am afraid that in the matter of Spanish dancing, we must depend upon Fanny Elssler or the two Noblett sisters (pl. 33). Dolores Seral (pl. 31),[1] who created such a vivid impression when she appeared, was one of the first to draw attention to the bold passion, perpetual grace and the supple voluptuousness characteristic of Spanish dancing, but she made no impression at all in Madrid; for Spaniards nowadays seem incapable of enjoying and understanding their own national dances. Whenever the jota aragonese or bolero is danced, the fashionable part of the audience rise and leave their seats and the only spectators left are the foreigners and persons of the lower classes in whom it is always more difficult to extinguish the poetic spirit.' The situation in the ballroom was apparently equally disappointing! 'Alas! they (the Spaniards) danced neither jota nor bolero, these dances being left to the servants, gypsies and peasants; but they danced quadrilles, rigadoons, and they waltzed. However, one evening, at our request, the two young ladies of the house offered to do the bolero, but before dancing, they took care to close the doors and windows of

[1]An Andalusian dancer famous in the early nineteenth century for her performance of the cachucha at the balls given at the Paris Opera House.

the patio, which were usually kept open, for they feared being accused of having bad taste, in liking local colour. Spaniards become angry when one mentions cachuchas, castanets, majos manolos, monks, smugglers and bullfighters, though in reality, they are very fond of all these truly national things. It should be remembered that we are speaking about the self-styled enlightened class inhabiting the cities.'

Baile nacional may not have been recognized by the smart set but, mercifully for posterity, the ordinary Spanish folk preserved it. The 'enlightened class' of city dwellers, referred to by Gautier, has expanded considerably since his day and their prejudices accordingly are more deeply ingrained and widespread than ever. It is quite common today to find these people proudly proclaiming their lack of expertize in the matter of Spanish dancing and continuing to look down on folklore or anything pertaining to it. Professional dancers they despise.

This long-standing prejudice is not really difficult to account for. During the nineteenth century, the effects of wars, political upheavals and rebellion within the country had almost completely deprived the Peninsula of first-class theatrical dancing. Instead of being in the hands of professional dancers, it fell into those of non-professionals who, whether they knew anything about dancing or not, jumped up on to platforms and performed in public as a means of earning easy money. People began to associate dancing in their minds with unskilled effort that was more than a little suspect. Ordinary Spaniards who worked hard for a living linked the dancers with nomads, gypsies and parasites who did not want to do a steady day's work. Dancing in public came to be regarded as anything but a profession, the people who performed were socially suspect and this prejudice, coupled with the unsettled state of the country, contributed to the steady decline in the quality of theatrical dancing and those who practised it. The curious paradox was that, at the same time, Spanish dancing was rising in favour outside Spain, rapidly becoming fashionable in foreign theatres where Spanish dancers were highly prized, and their dancing admired.

There was no doubt about the success of Spanish dancing enjoyed abroad, whatever the nineteenth-century Spaniard thought about his national dancing in his own land. It gained a footing in all the principal European opera houses, beginning with the Paris Opera House and extending through Central Europe to the Russian imperial theatres, and there it found a secure resting place. The ballet masters in Russia were quick to realize the theatrical possibilities of this unfamiliar form. More important still, they knew how to use it to the best advantage and, with highly-organized ballet companies at their disposal, were able to carry out their ideas. Under such favourable conditions it was not surprising to find many *assolutas* achieving the greatest successes of their careers through the medium of Spanish dancing and thereby influencing the taste of their audiences. Europe became the custodian of Spanish theatrical dancing at a time when it was plainly impossible for it to make much headway in the mother country.

The vogue for Spanish dancing abroad was due to a large extent to the personal success of Fanny Elssler, the famous Austrian ballerina. In 1830, she created a sensation in Paris, with her inspired performances of Spanish dances, accompanying herself on the castanets as she danced. Lithographs of the period have immortalized her for all time in her 'cachucha' costume (pl. 39). The critics never ceased to praise her when she performed suites of boleros, fandangos and cachuchas, and also her playing of the castanets impressed all who heard them. The notoriously difficult Parisian public applauded frantically every time her Spanish dances were presented, whether it was the novelty, or her own superb artistry that was responsible for this great success, will never be known, but certainly it was through this medium that she earned much of her fame. After the great Elssler had launched this particular type of dancing, many other dancers copied her, and henceforth Spanish dancing was highly esteemed in the leading theatres and was always to be found in the repertoires of the principal ballet companies.

The reigning queen at the Paris Opera House then was Marie Taglioni, who had taken Paris by storm with her sensitive interpretation of the romantic ballets. Fanny Elssler became her serious rival, so serious that the rivalry, becoming more and more intense, developed into a feud between the two famous ballerinas. So fierce did it become that opposite factions in the audience were formed

This controversy reminded one of that in Spain in the previous century when the relative merits of two other leading dancers were discussed and came under fire from two opposing groups.

Heated wrangling went on among the partisans of Taglioni and Elssler. The other worldliness of Taglioni's dancing transported her admirers to celestial heights and they never failed to acclaim her for the spirituality of her performances. Supporters of the 'divine' Elssler were carried away on to a totally different plane. They applauded the earthiness of her dancing, the vivacity and the passionate temperament she displayed in the performance of Spanish dances. She was dubbed 'the Spaniard from the North'! Hitherto, Taglioni had been famous for her stylization of national dances and perhaps, piqued by the success her rival obtained in the same field, she set the final seal of approbation on Spanish dancing in opera houses when she in turn took to playing the castanets and performing Spanish dances. The wings of the *sylphide* were shed and, succumbing to the joyous rhythms of the cachucha and similar dances, she became as successful as her rival in the same type of dancing. Taglioni danced *La Gitana* (pls. 40, 41) in 1838 at St. Petersburg and also at her farewell performance. Her castanets, together with her dancing slippers, have been preserved and may be seen at the Paris Opera House Museum.

Fame of a completely different kind was achieved by another foreigner, through the medium of Spanish dancing. It was difficult to understand why this person was so successful, because she was not really a professional dancer at all. Reputed to be Irish, but masquerading in turn as Sevillana, Madrileña, or Andalusian, she was professionally known as Lola Montes (pl. 42). She was never taken seriously as an artist but that did not prevent her going round the world performing Spanish dances. Wherever she went, she created a sensation, as much for the commotion she caused as for anything else, and soon her adventures received as much, if not more, publicity than her dancing.

In 1844, Lola Montes electrified the audience at the Paris Opera House by taking off a dancing slipper and hurling it at the head of a patron in the stalls because she was convinced that his presence brought her bad luck! That sort of behaviour did not earn for her

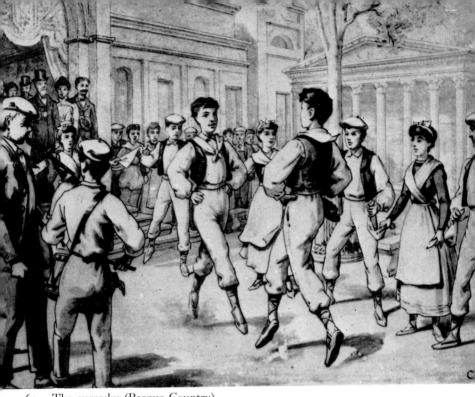

60. The aurresku (Basque Country).

61. La muneira (Galicia), open air version.

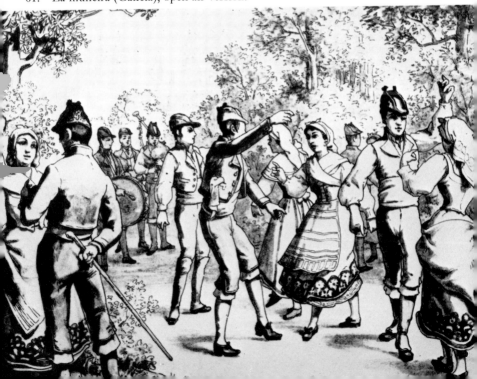

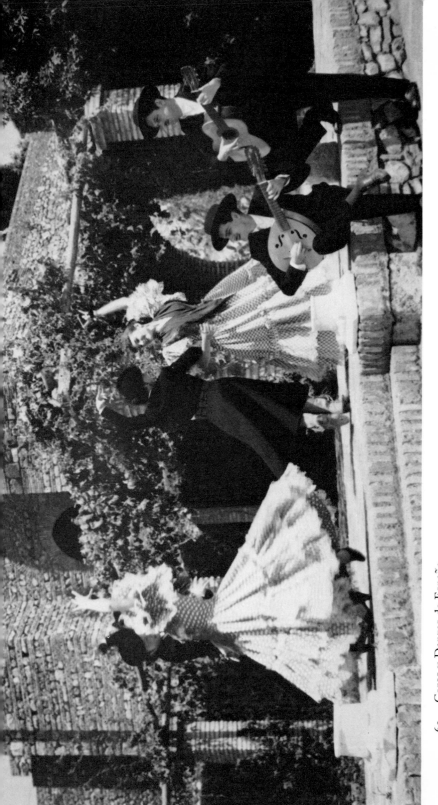

62. Coros y Danzas de España.

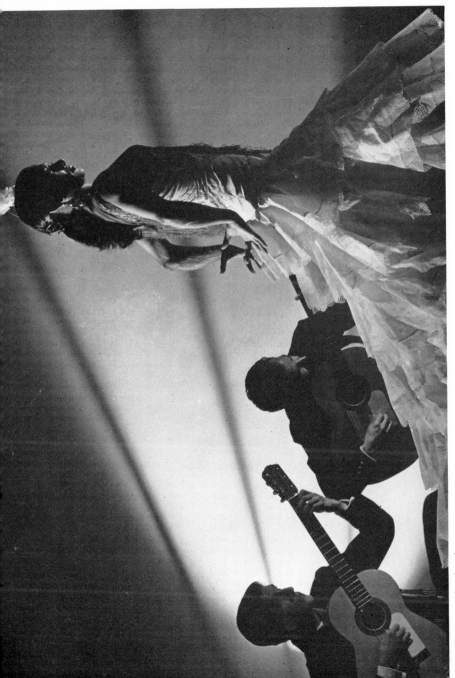

63. Flamenco in the theatre.

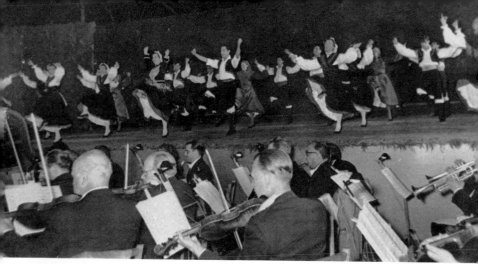

64. Antonio and Company in finale of the Galician Suite, taken during an open air performance in Vigo.

65. Stage version of the Galician Suite.

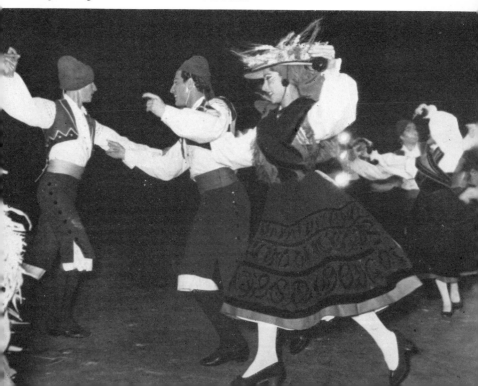

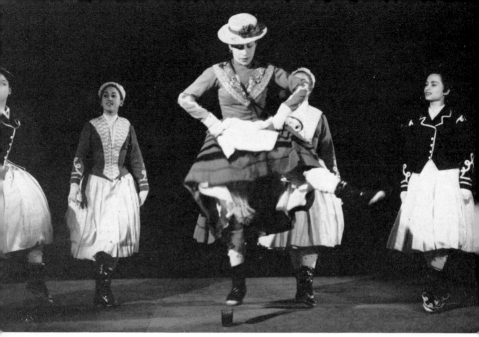

66.   Dancing on the tumbler; extract from Basque Suite.

67.   Suite of Basque dances, stage version.

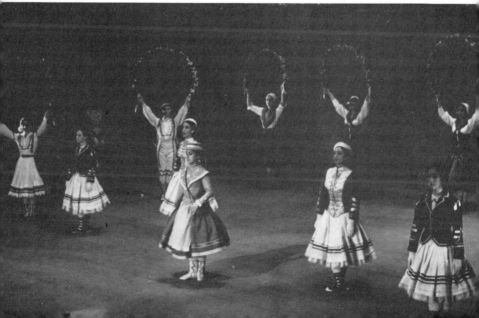

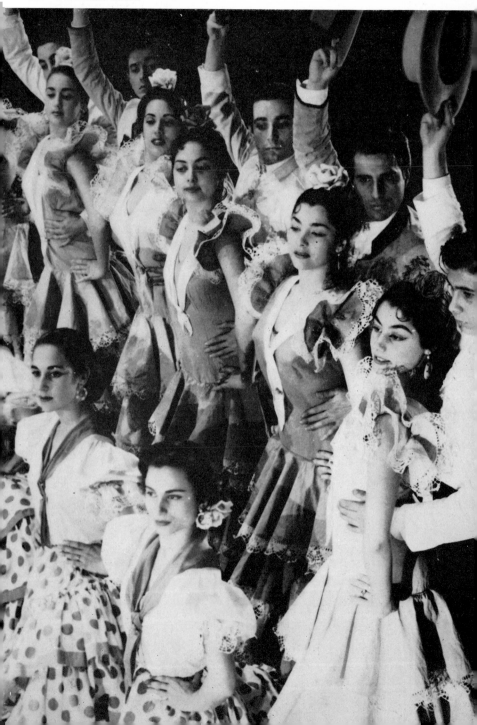

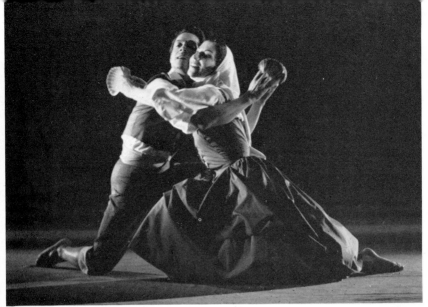

69. *Pas de deux* from Galician Suite; stage version by Antonio and Rosario.

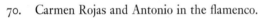

70. Carmen Rojas and Antonio in the flamenco.

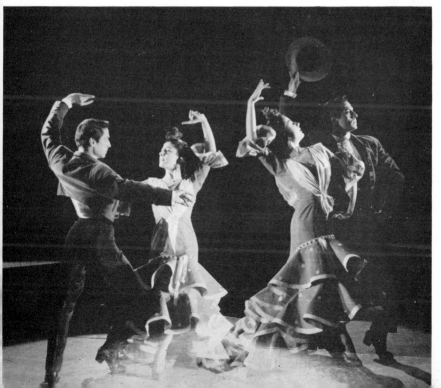

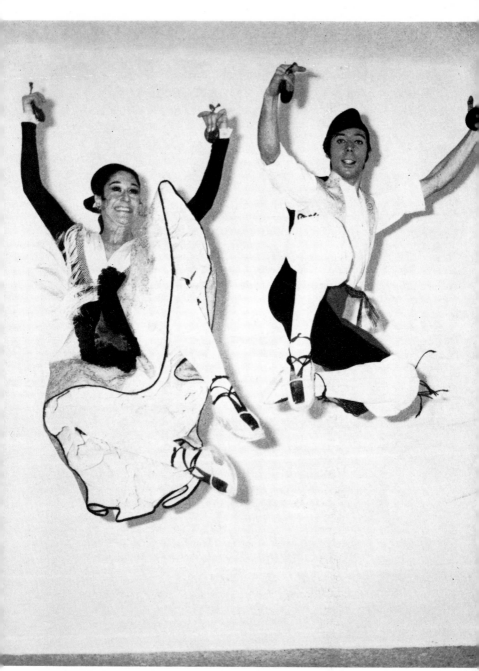

71. Maria Vejer and Enrique Burgos dance the Jota Aragonesa.

a very good reputation either in London or Paris, but this did not deter her from dancing in most of the other European opera houses and, as she went on her way, she popularized Spanish dancing abroad. Rulers of various states succumbed to her charms and she left a trail of bleeding hearts behind her. In Munich, she danced a cachucha and fandango at the Royal Theatre which brought forth simultaneous applause and hisses! Applauded presumably for her dancing, and hissed for the bad influence people thought she was having on Ludwig of Bavaria! The king had not evinced much interest in women before La Montes came on the scene. Lola Montes took herself very seriously indeed and danced her way into history. She wrote an irate letter to *The Times* in 1847 denying the charges made that her 'route had lain across a sovereign's heart'.

The type of Spanish dancing that was making such an impact upon foreign audiences at that time was unquestionably what was known as that of the Classical Bolero School. The first Spanish dancer reputed to have initiated French audiences into the pleasure of watching the native dances of Spain was Lola de Valencia (pl. 38). She also taught Fanny Elssler her famous cachucha. Too little is known about the instructors who were responsible for arranging the dances for the 'stars' of the romantic ballet period, which seems rather unfair considering how successful those artists were with their Spanish dances.

Apart from the performances of isolated Spanish dances, Spanish dance material was used profusely in the classical variations that were becoming a feature of nineteenth-century ballets. There was a growing tendency to blend different kinds of movement. This mixture of styles was intended to relieve the monotony of academic technique and, as such, was a continuation of the eighteenth-century desire to liberate the dances from the shackles of convention. As the choreographers of the period drew more and more upon Spanish material for this purpose, the success of the experiment led to Spanish dancing becoming a fashion in ballets which continued throughout the century.

Some of the ballets produced in the nineties became almost too overloaded with folk, national and character elements. One famous example was that of a variation containing no less than five distinct

11

influences: Spanish, Russian, Can-Can, Jig and Waltz! This stylization of Spanish solos became popular among both dancers and audiences; one has only to recall the delightful little bolero in the second act of *Coppelia* to observe how the material was adapted in France. Another novelty was flamenco on pointes and, in view of the mania for flamenco and ballet dancing today, one might expect a revival of this any minute now.

In Russia, the protagonist of this movement was Marius Petipa, a Frenchman who was fascinated by this sort of dance arrangement, and who did it very well. He was in Madrid in 1842 and in 1843 he partnered Marie-Guy Stephan at the Teatro del Circo (pl. 46). In the same year *Fleur de Granade* was produced in Spain; in 1844 *Perle de Seville*; in 1845 *Départ pour les Courses de Taureaux* and in 1846 *Carmen*. This visit profoundly influenced Petipa's later work, which was reflected in the profusion of Spanish dance steps he used in his full length classical ballets as, for example, *Swan Lake* or *Sleeping Princess*. The way in which he used Spanish dancing in his classical ballets proved how well-versed he was in this particular branch of dancing. He also enjoyed composing full length ballets on all-Spanish themes as, for instance, his *Don Quixote*, *Don Juan*, and *Paquita*. In the last named ballet he made his début in St. Petersburg as a dancer.

Petipa loved Spain and would have liked to settle there. He wanted to open a school in Madrid and offered his services to the authorities, but the offer was rejected because at the time it was thought that Spaniards had more serious things to think about than founding a national ballet school—an example of how history intervened to divert the current of Spanish dancing away from classical ballet in the Spanish theatre. Petipa finally settled in St. Petersburg, there to work with the Imperial Russian Ballet, and became the leading figure among the contemporary choreographers of that company. In time, his work became indissolubly associated with 'Russian Ballet'. How strange it seems now, that had it not been for the tragedy of war in Spain, that role might easily have been played there and he would nowadays be recognized as the nineteenth-century innovator of the Spanish ballet!

As if to prove to the world that though Spanish ballet appeared to be moribund in its own country, it was very much alive abroad, *Don Quixote* was produced in Moscow in 1869, then two years later in St. Petersburg. The libretto was by Petipa who probably based the ballet on that of the same name by Noverre in the previous century. *Don Quixote* by Petipa consisted of four acts and eight scenes. It was original in that it contained authentic Spanish steps which he had stylized—no doubt a gentle reminder of the time he had spent in Spain. This work alone would have guaranteed the survival of Spanish dancing on the international stage, but Petipa continued to compose numerous other full-length ballets on Spanish themes and a quantity of others with non-Spanish stories but including Spanish variations. By his creative imagination, Petipa did more than any other choreographer of his day to propagate Spanish theatrical choreography outside Spain.

Meanwhile, during all the time that dancers and ballet masters in the major European theatres were spreading protective wings over Spanish theatrical dancing, the situation continued to be serious in Spain. The country went through a protracted period of incessant strife; invasion, insurrection, even the dethronement of the monarchy. This was followed by more revolts, further political upheavals and only the restoration of the monarchy and the building of the Teatro Real brought about some semblance of artistic revival in the theatre (pls. 24, 30).

What then was the dance material available in Spain after these troublous times? Spain has been called the land of '*siestas* and *fiestas*' and, as has been observed, dancing was left in the hands of the people. The *fiestas* heading the list were undoubtedly those of a religious nature. These were a traditional necessity—war or no war —and no religious procession was complete without the appropriate dances. Next in favour came the *férias, romerías, verbenas, veladas, tertulias* and all the dancing in these was of a national nature. The open air was the natural background for this, whether in the intimacy of Andalusian patios or the public performances of plays on a larger scale, which were given in the plazas of the fine old Spanish cities. The balconies, draped with tapestries, shawls or oriental rugs, were the natural setting for the dances that were performed in the 'plaza'. They were also an essential part of the open-air plays known as 'verbenas'. The dancers swathed in Spanish shawls, with mantillas on their heads and high Spanish combs in their hair, undulated to the accompaniment of castanets and guitars. The boisterous crowd applauded them and more applause came from the balconies above from where the occupants of the houses were looking on. These entertainments, by contrast with the smaller intimate gatherings held in the patios of the south, were intended for large collective audiences and may still be seen from time to time.

Open-air festivals of music, singing and dancing were, and indeed still are an enjoyable feature of Spanish life. The dancers, singers and instrumentalists come from afar to compete with each other or, in the case of those of a local nature, on a more modest scale, from neighbouring hamlets and townships. It was a means of meeting friends, enjoying oneself generally and making propaganda for each particular region. These *bailes nacionales* were in the nature of 'mini' festivals and if it was very hot, or alternatively, in those parts of the country where the sun shines less and the rain comes down in torrents, the spectacles were held under canvas—either in tents or marquees, or with awnings slung across the squares suspended from the houses all round, as they are nowadays. The elements never prevented these functions from taking place.

Particularly in Andalusia, no *fiesta* was complete without dancing; that is to say, Andalusian dancing. Typical open-air bailes were given at night in the patios (pl. 43). Not without reason is Seville justly famous for her bailes and dance tradition; the Arabs discovered long ago that the climate lends itself to this kind of gathering. The inhabitants are born with an appreciation for dancing and they see it from infancy onwards. In the nineteenth century, the working class and gypsy quarters were the best places to find the nocturnal festivals known then as *bailes del candil* (pls. 44, 50) so called after the illumination that came from the *candiles*. A *candil* was a wick placed in a vessel filled with oil; these were placed in sconces on the walls of the patio, shedding a soft light upon the flowers, trees and swarthy faces of the spectators. The audience, consisting chiefly of artisans, bullfighters, gypsies and girls from the tobacco factory, was sometimes augmented by a few foreigners who might be lucky enough to find their way there, but generally these were popular entertainments rarely frequented by the upper classes.

Crowded into the small enclosure of the patio, the audience, helped along by the heat of the night, the endless 'canas' of manzanilla or sherry, or by the fiery fumes of aguardente, worked themselves up into a tremendous state of excitement as the concert proceeded—for this is what it really was. The guitarrists played, dexterously alternating thrumming on the soundboard of their guitars with their fingers and plucking the strings. Equally important were the 'cantaors' who intoned ancient ballads rarely heard elsewhere and who, in turn, were as indispensable as the dancers to the whole entertainment. There was little space at the disposal of the dancers and if necessary they did not hesitate to jump on to the tables to perform. Barefooted gypsy girls, male zapateadores and their audience were roused to a pitch of frenzy. Regarding the dancers appraisingly, gently puffing strong, aromatic black tobacco into the warm still atmosphere, the spectators completely lost themselves in the mood of the performance which was so arabic in feeling.

These gatherings were frequented by the real initiates; it was an enclosed world that no outside, disturbing influences would bother to penetrate. There were brief pauses in between the items and then little fish fried in oil, olives, anchovies and similar titbits were eaten. Then local gossip flowed, rather like a verbal newspaper with all the latest news from the bullring, praise or criticism of the performance, the current news from the tobacco factory and similar local founts of information. Pleasurable, warm, intimate evenings such as these, recalled those gatherings so beloved of the Moors in the same town, so very long ago.

The true habitat of traditional Spanish dancing in Spain, both in town and country, has always been the tavern, the café, or the inn where the local inhabitants are accustomed to gather. There, the people meet to relax and enjoy the good things of their land— Spanish music, Spanish dance, Spanish wine. At the period under review, the patriotic element was uppermost and so it is not surprising that *baile nacional* was the most popular.

Spain was war-weary; as one by one, she lost her colonies, the country became pervaded by a feeling of malaise and instinctively the people turned to everything local for comfort—something no foreigner could touch or take from them. Losing themselves in their native songs, ballads and dances, the people found the consolation they sought. Everybody had been through the same suffering and in the enjoyment of the simple arts of their own land they found a happy release from foreign intrusion and the tensions of war. To them, the songs and dances of Spain remained intact, they were living symbols representing a happier and more prosperous past and the people became very possessive in their attitude towards these art forms. They united the Spanish people in a way nothing else could for they had a deep meaning for them that no foreigner could hope to share.

In the intimate surroundings of the taverns and such like haunts (pl. 48), the depth of feeling expressed by the artists in their songs and dances created a warm rapport between the performers and the audience; whatever the mood, grave or gay, an atmosphere was created that would be difficult if not impossible to recapture in a large theatre. This kind of dancing was on a very personal level, understandable only to the initiated, for whom it was primarily intended.

A group of artists appearing in these popular places of entertainment was called a 'cuadro'. Usually there were about six performers taking part: guitarrists, dancers and singers. They sat on a tiny raised dais or small platform, or, if the tavern were too small even for that, a clearing was made on the floor for the dancers. When not performing themselves and awaiting their turn, the singers accompanied their companions as they danced with 'palmas', hand-clapping, 'pitos', finger snapping, 'palillos', castanets, or with tambourines. In a 'cuadro flamenco', the dances hailed from Andalusia—zorongos, canas, polos, jaleos, tiranas, malagueñas, and so forth. A verse of the song was sung by the dancer, generally expressing sentiments of a moving national, religious, or local nature, perfectly understandable to the local people present, but probably to nobody else. The dance followed and the 'cantaor', taking up the song with guitar accompaniment, joined the dancers who might be improvising. The musicians had to follow the dancers who accompanied themselves, while dancing, on the castanets. These items might be solos, duos or trios; space was limited and the dancers relied for effect upon violent footwork, flexible body movements, sinuous carriage of the arms and much facial expression. No technical *tours de force* such as ballet-lovers admire, for there was no space for those. The emotion was within the dancer, an individual evocation of sentiments expressed in movement and felt by the people assembled. It was at one and the same time a personal and collective experience in which every nuance of feeling was sensed. Gay or brooding, this kind of dancing referred to a past, a past common to all (pls. 51, 52).

Unable to contain themselves at times, the audiences were roused to wild enthusiasm, encouraging the dancers with signs of fellow-feeling, an occasional 'olé' of approbation, or, as the dance reached a climax, yells of delight, and this was the moment for everyone to join in, marking time by snapping their fingers, tapping their heels, clapping their hands or banging on the tables with empty glasses or bottles. As in the times of the Romans be it noted that all these pleasurable interludes were associated with the drinking of wine.

A 'cuadro' could be either 'flamenco' or 'bolero' and if the establishment were prosperous enough one of each might be engaged, but they were different and embraced two quite distinct styles of dancing. The 'cuadro bolero' was usually found in larger, less intimate functions which were held in *salones de fiestas*. These were large rooms similar to assembly rooms in England in the last century, and used for receptions, public dances and similar galas. A 'cuadro bolero' was generally engaged to entertain a large number of guests. In nineteenth-century Spain, dancing academies were sometimes hired for a similar purpose. The star attraction of the evening then was the appearance of a professional bolera and the rest of the programme was made up of items performed by the leading pupils from the *academia*. Rows of chairs were placed round the room and sometimes there was a gallery with portraits of local dancing celebrities adorning the walls. The prices of entrance varied, naturally those who paid most had the best seats, while those who paid next to nothing, had to stand throughout the evening.

The audience was mixed, ranging from the well-to-do to the man in the street and there were foreign visitors too.

Rattling castanets announced the arrival of the 'cuadro bolero'. They took up their positions and to the accompaniment of guitars, and playing castanets themselves, they embarked upon a lively, concerted number to open the proceedings. After that introduction came intricate variations of cachuchas, seguidillas, panaderos, fandangos and, of course, boleros, followed by separate or concerted items. Refreshments were served at a buffet and if a client invited a professional bolera to partake of something with him, the mother or elderly relative—who were then the customary chaperones—went too. This custom of taking mother or elderly relative still exists among Spanish dancers, only nowadays, the chaperone usually has to serve as dresser as well!

Returning to the theatre. No theatrical performance in Spain at that time ever concluded with anything other than an exhibition of *baile nacional*, whether play, opera, comedy or drama. Since the political situation was so unsettled, the theatres in Madrid only opened spasmodically, depending upon prevailing conditions. In the capital, the Principe presented drama; the Circo, acrobats and tumblers, zarzuelas, operas and ballets. Here it was that Petipa danced with the famous Spanish dancer of the time, La Fueco. The Lope de Vega Theatre gave plays or displays of *baile nacional* and these took up the whole evening. The Zarzuela Theatre also welcomed dance performances, but in all cases the dances had to tread the well-born path of tradition and were limited to one form of dancing only and that was *baile nacional*.

This was roughly the state of dancing in Spain at the time Queen Maria Christina came to the throne. A great lover of the arts, she founded the Conservatoire of Music in Madrid, and her husband, not to be outdone, responded by setting up a school for bullfighters in Seville. Nobody yet thought of opening a school of *baile nacional*, much less a ballet school!

When in 1849, Isabel II ascended the Spanish throne, a small theatre had already been attached to the royal palace in Madrid but only concerts were given there, either of operatic or sacred music. To herald the royal marriage, a series of artistic festivals were given during the entire week before the wedding. Grand displays of *baile nacional* took place in the open air—which the bride attended—and the plays invariably concluded with *baile nacional*.

During Isabel's reign spasmodic attempts were made to continue work on the original building of the projected opera house. By a strange coincidence, every attempt seemed to be thwarted by some major national disaster. There was still a feeling that Madrid without an opera house was not a real capital city and could not take her place by the side of the other European capitals already possessing one. Headed by the queen herself, a meeting was convened to discuss the matter, and finally it was decided that the opera house must be completed without further delay (pl. 53). This was a very auspicious moment, for it happened to coincide with the streets of Madrid being lit by gaslight and also the laying of the first railway lines.

Built on the original site of the Teatro de los Caños del Peral, the opera faced the main entrance of the royal palace and was five storeys high. The Spanish people had waited a long time for their theatre, which they now regarded with pride as the finest in Europe and more beautiful than any other in the world. Once opened, and in spite of events in the last century, it was soon given up to the production of Italian opera. This necessitated elaborate ballets but there was still no sign of any organized training school and it is not made very clear where the dancers came from. Musicians and singers were still being prepared at the Conservatoire and so there was an excellent orchestra and a very good chorus at the Opera House.

We know that there was a ballet company comprising sixty boys and girls and it was suggested that these might form the nucleus of the long projected ballet school but nothing came of this plan either. Like that of 1807, it proved to be abortive. Although the works presented at the Opera House were Italian, the ballet group was Spanish and there was a tendency to resist foreign infiltration there. Most of the soloists, however, were from abroad. Fanny Elssler, Emma Livry, La Cerrito, had all appeared at one time or another. It would appear from this, that it was the absence of training facilities that necessitated bringing in the foreign ballerinas.

Let a Spanish writer describe the conditions under which young Spanish dance artists were expected to grow and develop:

A rheumaticky old ballet mistress, swathed in wraps and mufflers, swished her little cane across the legs of her pupils, who, for the most part, were sad, anaemic and stupid. Like a lot of beggars, shivering with cold, huddled into corners with their frozen hands tucked under their armpits and with arms crossed over their hollow little chests, they followed the harpy's invocations with the impassivity of a herd. All their misery and sadness was reflected in the smallest step or the most insignificant position they took. A member of the Opera *corps de ballet* was a disturbing and horrifying sight. Against this background of bewildered, roughened human beings, stood out by contrast, the heavy-calved ballerina, who had not the faintest idea of line, plastic movement or anything else—except 'pointes' and similar nonsense. The *corps de ballet* was fodder for the lecherous old men who, like villains in a play, twirling their moustaches, went to the 'Redondilla' to invite the dancers to steak and chips in a private room at 'Fornos'[2] or else, maybe not even steak and chips.

This extract, taken from Mathilde Munoz's *Historia del Teatro Real* paints a rather grim picture and makes it sound as though it was not much fun to be at the Real. The unfortunate nineteenth-century ballet girl in Spain had a wretched life, nothing glamorous about it, nor anything remotely aesthetic about the meagre instruction she received. The reader can only marvel that anyone ever reached the status of soloist—heavy-calved or otherwise. The scathing references to pointe work are interesting and make it obvious that this was not an aspect of balletic technique that was very highly esteemed at the Royal Opera House. How the dancers were ever elevated to the 'pointage' is very mysterious, considering that they had no adequate preparation. Why was the governing body apparently so disinterested in the artistic education of their young dancers and so indifferent to their welfare?

There is some enigma here. In most cases, if there is no instructional establishment attached to a national company it is because there are no funds available, but this was not the case at the Real, had they wanted a school. The degrading conditions under which the dancers were expected to live and work suggests that this lack might be connected with the prejudiced idea that young dance

[2]Famous restaurant in Madrid.

artists should not be in any way cultivated—an idea still prevalent today. This was very different from royal establishments elsewhere at the same period, where dancers were trained in the same way as musicians and given the opportunity of cultivating the graces of life, and thus fitting them to take their places in the social pattern of court life.

The status of a ballet dancer was considerably lower than that of other artists at the Real. The *corps de ballet* received smaller salaries than the chorus in the opera and were considered to be of minor importance from every point of view. Ballet girls in those days were expected to amuse any old roué who took a fancy to them. In the Opera House, there was a room, circular in shape and therefore known as the Redondilla. This served the purpose of a 'green room' and there, the ballet girls, tricked out in their tutus, arrived to meet their beaux. Radiant or not as the case might be, they received their escorts and their presents in the Redondilla. The gentlemen of the town, armed with champagne, boxes of sweets with tiny waxen dolls on the lid, were there, all prepared to make their amorous overtures. If the girl was lucky, she might find a jewelled trinket hidden in the flowery depths of her bouquet but that is as far as pecuniary success went. Unlike the singers, dancers rarely made fortunes from this sideline; they had to be content with wining, dining, or riding in the carriages of the wealthy. As for the poor male dancer, he remained in his dressing-room after the performance, uncourted hungry and despondent.

How astonishing it is to find that in Spain, the most formal of lands, nothing was done to prepare dancers attached to the Royal Ballet for this most arduous and exacting profession! It is still more amazing to find that they had little choice in their private lives either. It was no honour to belong to the *corps* at the Real, closely resembling, as it did, the oldest profession in the world. It might be thought that here was something for the moralists to really thunder about—traditionally so verbose in Spain, when morality applied to dance and dancers was in question, but as far as this subsidized national temple of art was concerned, they remained strangely silent. It can be imagined what a nightmare it was for those directing these rough, untrained dancers. It is recorded that they 'had to impose their authority in order to maintain discipline'.

The first company at the Opera House consisted of an unspecified number of principals, who may have been guest artists. They were supported by three second dancers, one coryphée and three extras, three mime artists and a *corps de ballet* of twenty-eight. The male section of the group consisted of three first dancers, three mime artists and a *corps de ballet* of twenty-four. To these male and female artists must be added the sixty boys and girls already mentioned. The ballet master was also the choreographer, and he had one assistant.

Small credit was accorded to the choreographers then. There was apparently no Spanish 'Domingo Rossi' forthcoming in the nineteenth-century Spanish theatre. How could there be? The poor ballet masters probably had so many jobs to do, training the dancers in addition to everything else, that they had no time left for any creative work. Yet, there must have been some young prospective Spanish choreographers in their midst, capable of designing Spanish ballets, had they been given the chance and suitable working conditions. The Italian and French companies had left a model on which to work and it was reasonable to expect that now, with a magnificent theatre, Spanish ballet in the grand manner could go right ahead. Outside Spain, Petipa was demonstrating how beautifully Spanish dancing could be fitted into the framework of classical ballet. Inside Spain, from the Royal Opera House, no full length Spanish ballets emerged, no suites of ancient Spanish dances were brought up to date, nothing startling or original was produced. The ballet masters appeared to have no choice, other than to depend on the repertory of foreigners, and to string together sequences of well-known Spanish steps.

The direction did not seem to have any choreographic policy whatever, making it quite impossible for the ballet to do anything other than stagnate. No training school for the dancers meant no suitable material for a native choreographer to work on; an intolerable situation from an artistic standpoint. The stage of the Real was no place to experiment and the building therefore never became the shrine of national art in Spain it was intended to be. So much effort had been expended but from a Spanish point of view it was Dead Sea fruit by the time it came into existence. What should have been of inestimable value was the gift of Italian opera and ballet to Spain, but instead, most Spanish artists had little heart for this impersonal and un-Spanish form of art. The Real was the target for perpetual criticism from the press, mainly because it was subsidized. That was not all, for though the situation resembled that of the previous century, the cause of acrimony this time was not only foreign artists it was also the unfair way of spending the subsidy that infuriated people. If it were true that money was being showered upon this expensive form of foreign art, why could not the government do something similar for the theatre sponsoring Spanish works? The Zarzuela Theatre, seating over two thousand people, was still producing all-Spanish works but received nothing, while the Real did. Why? This was the bone of contention.

The Spanish people adored the zarzuelas for their gaiety, national themes, and national dances accompanied by catchy tunes. One of the most successful in the nineteenth century was that with an English missionary as the leading comic figure. He lived with the gypsies in order to learn their language and the fun that ensued in the dialogue may be imagined. The Englishman kept popping on and off the stage trying out his execrable 'gypsy' Spanish. This was probably a skit on George Borrow and to us has a distinctly Gilbert and Sullivan flavour.

In spite of the popularity of zarzuelas, the theatre presenting them ran at a loss, due it was claimed, to the crippling overhead expenses. The Real, exempt from taxation, was close by, giving only foreign works and making a handsome profit. When these unfortunate facts were revealed, there was a flood of protest. The eminent musicologist Ansejo Barblere published an article on the subject in 1877 saying: 'When one sees in Spain, that we have the celebrated Zarzuela Theatre where the genius of Spanish artists is born and developed, maintained by the generosity of thousands of private individuals and industry, yet, the Government does not even cast a protective glance in its direction, one may fairly exclaim: "enough of irritating privilege, equal justice for all".'

As a result of this exposure, a leading newspaper published an article comparing the expenditure involved in the upkeep of the two theatres. This revealed that the Real, while enjoying the use of the theatre, paid no rent, while the Zarzuela paid not only a high rental, but also taxes! The Real which concerned itself only in featuring foreign artists, was compared with the Zarzuela which only sponsored Spanish works. The losses suffered by the Zarzuela were compared with the profits made by the Opera House. More comparisons were made between the small salaries paid to the Zarzuela artists with those at the Real. The final sensational news was that the impresarios earned more money than all the artists put together! In making these revelations to the public, the writer made it clear that he was personally opposed to all subsidies in principle and therefore did not wish to see the Zarzuela subsidized; he felt very strongly, however, that it was iniquitous to support foreign art when it was at the expense of the Spanish artists and to their detriment.

He added: 'The Real is a state theatre, built with national money, yet, complete with all its commodities, any impresario is permitted to exploit it and this, today, when we are threatened with new taxes. Because subsidies are accepted in theory by everyone, no court or newspaper is disposed to criticize this generosity. Why then are not all theatres proportionately subsidized?' His final despairing salvo was: 'I am sure there will be no satisfactory answer forthcoming to my question. We are in Spain.'

The protests dragged on interminably. Right until the end of the century echoes of the controversy about the Real still resounded.

There were many people who patronized the theatre who were not so interested in opera or ballet as in being seen at the Royal Opera House. It was smart to go and gave them something to talk about. Foreign works by Rossini, Handel, Glück and many other famous composers of the day were performed regularly.

In the present century, the brilliant seasons of international opera and ballet continued and were as much part of the social round in Madrid as they were at the same period in London or Paris. In 1914, Diaghleff arrived with his company, and to mention Stravinsky's name then was synonymous with 'Russian Ballet'. Nyjinsky danced in *Scheherezade*, *Firebird*, *Carnaval*, *Les Sylphides*, and *Petrouchka*. King Alfonso XIII never missed a single performance when the incomparable Anna Pavlova danced at the Real. The Royal Opera House ran true to form right up to the end of its existence, in that foreign works were exclusively performed there. In 1925, the doors closed, as most Spaniards then thought—for ever.

After the Civil War, a tentative effort was made to reopen the Real, but it was quickly closed again when, during a performance, the audience in the stalls had the unusual experience of finding their feet in water! Unexpectedly a rivulet had gushed into the theatre and down the aisles of the stalls! All sorts of reasons were given to account for this. Underground boring connected with the construction of the Metro was blamed for disturbing the subterranean currents. Going back to history, when Philip II moved the capital to Madrid in 1561, his counsellors did not think of telling him that Madrid stood on ground beneath which flowed underground currents, liable to spring up unexpectedly in unpredictable places. Had they done so, it might have been foreseen that water could not be very far from the theatre since the original edifice was built on the site of a fountain that later became the wash-houses of the Caños del Peral and the theatre bearing the same name!

The Ministry of Education succeeded in obtaining a grant of six million pesetas to reopen the theatre once more, but until quite recently it remained closed, and people asked in vain the reason. The romantically minded Madrileños saw in it a dreaming figure of the past; the more brutally outspoken called it a 'chronic nightmare'. To lovers of Spanish dancing it is a living monument commemorating former triumphs from the time when it was the birthplace of Spanish ballet. Recently, the Real has been reopened and is now used as a concert hall.

Whatever may happen in the future, it should not be forgotten that on this site ballet in Spain in the international sense was first fostered. It was in the Caños del Peral in the eighteenth century that early experiments in the development of ballet as an art form took place. There it was that foreign dance influences were incorporated into a developed Spanish theatrical dance-form. Reopening its doors in the nineteenth century as the Royal Opera House, it became a centre for foreign dancers who, on returning home, interpreted Spanish dancing to international audiences. By the end of the century, most of the world-famous dancers and chore-ographers of their day had appeared there.

So much for the past and now, what is happening to Spanish theatrical dancing? So far, our chief concern has been with Spanish dancing with reference to its influence in the theatre. Little has been said about that popular aspect of Spanish dancing known as 'regional' or 'folk' and still less about 'flamenco'. Now that there is so much discussion about the national theatre that it is planned to build in the modern part of Madrid, the time has come to review the Spanish dance material at present available, and also to consider its effect upon the audiences of the present day, and how they in their turn are slowly transmuting it into yet another form—still bearing national characteristics, but not always quite within the limits of what was hitherto considered to be a Spanish framework.

8

National Dance and the Influence of Flamencomania

THE COLLECTIVE term *baile nacional* was extensively used in the last chapter and the time has come to examine this *baile nacional* or, 'national dance', and see what it consists of. In the past, the word 'baile' was used in Spain to denote dancing of a regional and folk nature, usually performed for and by the people.

In those days, Spaniards associated *baile nacional* with 'folk' as opposed to 'stage' dancing. Nowadays, the one has been merged with the other. Rarely, if ever, is Spanish dancing now performed before a selective Spanish audience as it was in the past, as a gesture of national pride and independence. In modern dress, Spanish dance now gives pleasure to a much wider public, spread all over the world, who go to see it because they like it. As of old, the dances still consist of solos, duets, trios or of larger groups of dancers. Relics of the old, popular, social dances are still to be found in this hybrid form of theatrical dance, usually as a rollicking rumbustuous finale to the programme, with all the dancers joining in. The most varied Spanish dances are still those called 'regional'. These dances are as diverse as the languages spoken in Spain and for the same reason—they are racially distinct.

As everyone knows, the official language spoken in Spain is Castilian, but that does not prevent the Catalans speaking Catalan, the Galicians Gallego, or the Basques retaining their own Basque language. In the same way as Gaelic is spoken by Irish, Scottish and Welsh inhabitants in Great Britain and differs from English, so it is in Spain, only on a much larger scale. A foreigner may well wonder at times how Spanish are the regions? Every Spaniard I met seemed to be imbued with an almost mystic love of the earth upon which he was born. A man from Oviedo is convinced that only the Asturias counts and that there is no more lovely spot in Spain than his 'patria chica'. A native of Seville will go further and maintain that unless you were born in Seville you could not be Spanish! North, south, east and west, it is all Spain but, apart from the fact that all the inhabitants are Spanish, they cling to their own race, language and customs, and it is precisely their songs and dances that help them to maintain their much prized individuality and this is part of the urge for racial self-preservation.

Since times are changing, life in the Spanish regions is no longer quite the same and local customs are being adapted to new conditions. The meaning of Spanish dance changes, as it does elsewhere incidentally, according to the period and place in which it is performed. Regional life is speeding up, so is the tempo of the dances —in many cases to please the relatively new public, who can now enjoy the fruits of modern standards of technique, as entertainment is relayed to them by means of television and travel abroad. These innovations are bound to make inroads upon the Spanish preconceived national standards of living, which are becoming less and less tenable. Local colour is beginning to fade, even some of the caves of Sacromonte have vanished; many of the gypsies who lived there have been rehoused and, abandoning their native, distinctive mode of dressing, live like the rest of the world. Those who remain in their caves are as much a tourist attraction as anything else. Nevertheless, despite their changing world, they still manage to hold on to the traditions of their race in some things as, for example, in holding their annual competitions. These take place in Andalusia with the intention of electing the best gypsy artists from among the dancers, singers and guitarrists of their race. A first prize went in recent years to a 'cantaor' for his rendering of an ancient ballad recounting a thirteenth-century Spanish victory in battle, handed down to him from his grandfather.

Tastes may change as modern standards seep into the regions, but so far, the individual style of dancing peculiar to each region has been retained and the local form of dance is carefully preserved.

Before discussing the actual content of Spanish dance material, it might be as well to mention in passing that it is not only the changing social conditions within Spain that are responsible for modifying the dances of the country, it is also the demands made by the ever-expanding audiences abroad whose taste can be immediately perceived by the box office returns! It would be useless to present to a cosmopolitan flamencomaniac audience the sort of Spanish dance foreigners used to enjoy not so many years ago. It consisted of a sultry Spanish lady with a carnation between her teeth and a stiletto tucked into her garter! Nowadays this would be treated by *aficionados* as a huge joke or even a caricature of non-Spanish (meaning flamenco of course) origin.

Audiences, on the other hand, are in their turn influenced by what they see on the stage. In recent years, it has become fashionable for governments to send out highly-specialized groups of dancers, specially trained for the purpose and permanently employed to show their *baile nacional* to the world. Usually large, these companies require stadiums or big theatres for their rallies where they compete for such accolades as 'the most spectacular company in the world'. A far cry indeed from the old conception of national dancing as a spontaneous means of expression of the people and, still less, that of a simple form of recreation for the peasants. If Spain has only succumbed to this fashion on a relatively modest scale, it is possibly because she has no subsidized national theatre to provide these spectacular groups. Most Spanish companies are privately owned and controlled. They do present some very spectacular suites of regional dances which are now to be seen quite as frequently on the stage as they used to be in their natural habitat, the countryside or open town squares. Let us now turn our attention to the content of this dance material which in recent years has become so popular on the stage and in certain cases, highly profitable.

Spanish dances are identifiable by their geographical demarcation. Spain consists of fifty provinces overlapping each other. Each district within a province prides itself upon the local variation of the basic regional dances. To a casual observer, a dance from a certain region may resemble that from the neighbouring one so much as to be indistinguishable. Dialect in language is recognized, but is not so well-known when applied to dancing. In England it would be difficult for any but the expert to differentiate between the nuances of accents in adjoining counties; likewise in Spanish regional dancing, only a specialist could assess the degree of dance influence exerted from one region to another, close by. For those who would like detailed information on this subject, the admirable series of books by Garcia Matos[1] are available. This folk-lorist has devoted his life to serious research and is in the process of working through the dances of Spain, region by region. It is not the purpose of this chapter to give an exposition on this matter, but rather to indicate a general outline of the type of dances, regional in origin, that are taking root in the theatre today and making Spanish dancing famous there, throughout the world.

For the sake of brevity, the dances may be divided into four basic groups; from the north, the south, the east and the west. From the north come the jotas; from the south, the fandangos; from central and western Spain, the seguidillas; from the east, the sardanas. Two other categories of dances will have to be considered separately, namely those of the Basques and those belonging to the Spanish gypsies. Nearly all the Spanish dancing seen in the theatre nowadays belongs to one or more of these groups and the dances themselves consist of ramifications of one or other of these basic types. The dances are highly stylized and a taste for stylization is increasing. The influence the theatre is exerting upon this once spontaneous expression of the Spanish dancers is liable to become stronger as the establishment of a permanent theatre in Madrid ceases to be a subject of discussion and becomes a reality.

Dealing with the jota first. This dance, affectionately termed the 'father of Spanish dances' by the Spaniards, is typical of the north. The origin of the jota is obscure although theories on the subject are not lacking. Spanish authorities on the subject differ in their opinions. Some claim it is Greek in origin and others that it is Arabic. The grounds for this theory seem to be that the Arabs were in possession of Zaragoza from the eighth until the beginning of the twelfth century, and their influence endured until the

[1]Garcia Matos: *Danzas Populares de España*. Madrid, Sección Feminina de F. E. y de Las J.O.N.S. 1957.

seventeenth century when the Moriscos were finally expelled from Spain. A third school of thought claims that the jota is not an ancient dance, but belongs at the earliest to the seventeenth century, if not the eighteenth. The latter conviction is reinforced by the fact that the earliest reference to it being performed in a theatre did not appear until the eighteenth century, when Ramon de la Cruz mentioned it in one of his plays. This may only apply to the theatrical version of the dance and does not exclude the possibility of the popular version having been danced before that time.

The accepted home of the jota is Aragon (pl. 54) and Navarre (pl. 55), but something very like it is danced everywhere in Spain. It is alleged to have come to Aragon from Valencia but when, why, or how, remains a mystery. In days gone by, it was used for curative purposes much in the same way as the tarantella was in Italy. Nowadays it is danced at popular gatherings, both secular and sacred. As is the case in most dances from northern Spain, which are more boisterous than those from the south, the jota slackens in tempo as it travels towards the Mediterranean coast. The steps of the dance are performed on the ball of the foot, the angle of the foot varies, sometimes being turned in, out, or at times kept quite straight. Nowadays, it is danced in rope-soled slippers called 'alpagartas'; illustrations in the last century indicate that the women danced it in bare feet. Rhythmically, it is in triple time and the rapid footwork includes toe and heel movements, stamping of the feet, high springing steps for the men, lower for the women, and there are also beaten steps. Both sexes perform movements of a crouching nature, consecutively kneeling first on one knee with great velocity, then on the other, followed instantly by swift leaps into the air. Rapid, varied movements of this kind require flexible ankle and knee joints and strong thigh muscles. The steps often appear to be executed just a little after the beat, resulting in a lilting effect of great charm, caused by the counter-rhythm in the music and is rather like a tiny rhythmic hiccup, very characteristic of the jota. It is not necessary to cover a lot of ground in this dance, the dancers perform almost on one spot. What is important, is neatness of footwork combined with perfect timing, and syncopation is typical. The jota demands technical facility and muscular strength to achieve the requisite speed. To perform this dance adequately, a good musical sense and natural feeling for the rhythm are indispensable. By comparison with dances from other Spanish regions, head, body and arm movements are used sparingly. Tambourines, mandolines, guitars and other plucked instruments of the same family, together with the human voice and castanets, provide the musical accompaniment for the dance.

Leaving the north and travelling through Old and New Castile, La Mancha and as far west as Extremadura, the seguidillas becomes the type dance (pl. 56). There can be no doubt about the antiquity of the seguidillas. Writers before Cervantes referred to it. Writing in the sixteenth century, Mateo Aleman cited the seguidillas when discussing changing fashions to illustrate his point. He explained that buildings, weapons, furniture, games, music and dancing all changed in the course of time and selected the seguidillas as an example. Since this dance had replaced the sarabande, he remarked that it was only a question of time before the seguidillas in turn would be replaced by something else.

The seguidillas originally came from Don Quixote's country, La Mancha. Like many other Spanish dances, it was primarily a song and the Manchegos regarded it as the quintessence of Spanish dancing. The performers took up their positions to the strumming of the guitar, but did not move immediately; the guitar continued playing and the singers sang a verse. Only then, did the dancers give a roll on the castanets as a signal that they were about to dance. After dancing the first copla (or verse) the dancers suddenly stopped dead still, quite deliberately, for this was an outstanding feature of the dance. The guitars played on without ceasing for an instant, and the dancers, accompanying themselves on the castanets, only started to dance again after a very long pause, while the singers and guitarrists went on with their playing and singing. The music played on and this process of stopping abruptly on the part of the dancers continued again and again. There was nothing accidental about these pauses, they were carefully contrived, for, to stop suddenly and at the same time, gracefully, required great skill, so it was thought. This all-important pause was called the 'bien parado'. Now obsolete, it is rarely seen in the modern version of the dance.

The seguidillas, like the jota, penetrated other regions, each one having a special local variation of the dance. The best known abroad is the one from Seville known as the sevillanas. Usually danced by couples in heeled shoes, it contains light springing steps but without any of the 'jig' quality peculiar to northern dances. Everything is smooth in this dance and this smoothness of movement is emphasized in the sevillanas by the beautifully co-ordinated sinuous use of the arms, shoulders and body. This is particularly noticeable in the crossing steps when the dancers change places with each other. The elegance of the shoulder movement is reminiscent of the eighteenth-century 'shading' of the shoulders typical of the early French minuets. Inclined from the waist, the body gently turns forwards, backwards or in a lateral direction; a subtle movement never in any way exaggerated. Half and whole turns combined with hip movements, light stamping of the feet and flowing movements from the upper part of the body are all typical of the sevillanas. The footwork has to conform to the carefully balanced rhythmic pattern of the music and the ground patterns are extremely varied. This is a dance that need not depend upon spectacular leaps into the air for effect, or crashing down on to the knees; on the contrary, almost feline, flowing movements proceeding from the waist upwards combined with strong footwork, hammering out the complex rhythms and counter-rhythms, are its salient features. As might be expected, the accompaniment is similar to that of the seguidillas; song, guitar and castanets.

The measure and balance of this dance is assured by the arrangement of steps into set coplas; each copla takes up an equal amount of music, always returning to a refrain, identical each time in rhythm and design. As in the old seguidillas, the dancers pause between the coplas, in order to gather strength for the next one, because, as the dance proceeds, each successive copla becomes faster as it contains more steps than the previous one, that have to be fitted into the same musical pattern. Arms, head, and body movements are harmoniously blended with those of the feet.

The sevillanas has been called the 'mother' of Spanish dancing in the same way that the jota was identified as the 'father'. Time has proved that these two dances are a magnificent source for theatrical choreography. The sevillanas in particular, while adhering to a set form, is flexible, for it can be varied from the very simple to the very intricate, depending upon the virtuosity of the dancers. The quality of the dance is determined by the conditions under which it is performed; in the ballroom, theatre, cabaret or in the open air at the Feria de Sevilla. Wherever this dance is found it is always conspicuous by the purity of its form.

Penetrating deeper into Andalusia, we find in the south that the typical dance is the fandango (pl. 57). Many Spaniards consider this to be the earliest of all Spanish dances but opinions differ on this matter too. The fandangos, like the seguidillas, adhere to a set form, consisting of coplas. The length of these coplas depends upon those of the song accompanying the dance. First, the copla is danced, followed by a refrain of set steps to which the dancers constantly return at the end of each copla. The fandango is danced at a brisk pace, sometimes working up to a frenzy at the end especially, as so often happens, when it is the concluding item on a programme. It is in triple time, the steps contain many heel beats, known as 'taconéo'; these beats are combined with complicated rhythmic patterns on the castanets. When the feet are still, the movement is transferred to the wrists, undulating with the arms and hips. Fandangos are performed in heeled shoes, the movements are close to the ground and the further south one goes, this earthiness becomes more marked. One of the attractive features of this dance is the manner in which the girls use their skirts, usually of vivid colours. The dance is transformed into a kaleidoscope of movement and colour as, at the climax, everything appears to be moving; staccato beats of the feet, play of the castanets, continuous manipulation of the head, body and arms, all in unison with the voluminous skirts. The movement seems to travel into space, right through the wrists and fingers. An exciting dance to watch, it is one of the most popular and, like the sevillanas, may still be seen in the streets, taverns and such caves as are left in Andalusia. This ancient folk-dance loses none of its inherent strength, power and virility when removed from the natural surroundings in the open air and has been most successfully transplanted into the theatre.

The fourth group of dances to be considered are those from the east, in Catalonia, which may be extended to include Valencia. These dances are of a very different nature from those just mentioned. The Greeks occupied this coast in the past and remains of their culture are still to be seen in the dances there. Evidence of this influence are at once apparent in the prevalence of linked circle dances of the 'kola' type, frequently found among the people on the Mediterranean coast. Another point of interest in the dances from this region, is the survival of elements from the old aristocratic dances which have become incorporated into the popular dances. These are noticeable in the ceremonial entrances consisting of honours and movements of courtesy, with which so many Catalonian and Valencian dances commence. These would appear to stem from the Middle Ages and are a reminder of the close links formerly maintained between the courts of Provence and Barcelona.

The best known dance is the Catalan sardana which is a round dance. Another, less famous abroad, is the contrapás, a linked dance composed of skipping steps. There is also the ball plá based on steps of the 'pas de Basque' family, only with the feet not turned out as in the classical variety. According to legend, the sardana was originally for ladies only and men were forbidden to enter the circle; the men in revenge danced the contrapás and women were not permitted to join in with them. Finally, all came to an amicable understanding and both sexes participated in both dances.

The Catalans claim that the farandole came from the contrapás but there does not appear to be anything to support this claim; it is far more probable that the farandole, which was the type dance of Provence, came to Catalonia with the Provençal court in the thirteenth century since when it has been adopted by the Catalonian people.

One of the most pleasant sights to be seen in Catalonia is that of the people dancing the sardana (pl. 58), not only in the villages, but in the capital city as well. Go to the Cathedral Square in Barcelona on Sunday morning, and there you will find mixed groups of people both old and young, Spanish as well as foreign, treading a measure together with obvious enjoyment. The dance is the sardana, belonging to the branle circle type for 'as many as will' and it is danced to the accompaniment of high-pitched pipes and percussion instruments. The rule is that nobody may be refused permission to join the circle of dancers. It does not matter in the least whether the newcomers know the dance or not. A circle may start with a couple of dancers and grow, as more and more people are tempted from the watching crowd to join in. The same fundamental steps are performed in all the groups, but how different is the mode of dancing them! One circle may consist of experts who, meeting regularly, are very sure of what they are doing. They may even be rehearsing for some local competitions which are still a feature of Catalan life. Dancing in this context is a serious business and the dancers are seen to be concentrating on the careful placing of each step, at exactly the same moment as their neighbour and always keeping at an even distance from each other. These are not professional dancers but probably students from the university whose performance might be compared with that of any well drilled *corps de ballet*. They allow nothing to divert their attention; not even the yells from the noisy crowd disturb them. The dancers are all dressed alike, in white, including their rope-soled 'alpagartas' and this, as they step with the utmost care and precision, adds to the great feeling of uniformity this performance gives to the onlooker.

The circle revolves slowly and tends to render the dance monotonous but it is of a restful, tranquilizing kind of monotony, as the sustained gyratory movements, endlessly performed in a clockwise circle, exert a strangely hypnotic effect upon one. The interesting contrast lies in the sudden change of tempo and pitch of the music for the 'cortos' and 'largos' which constitute this dance. The former, smoothly danced with the arms down by the dancers' sides, and the latter, lightly springing steps with the arms raised above the shoulders, but always holding the hands of the dancers on either side. The Catalans belong to a serious-minded race and this state of mind is reflected in the solemnity of this kind of Catalan dance which is sharply contrasted with the performances of the dancers in the other mixed groups.

These come from every part of the globe and are obviously out to enjoy themselves. Straggling along, they follow the Catalans as best they can; laughing, talking, or maybe yelling, to make themselves heard above the shrill tones of the pipes. The pattern of the dance is barely discernible in this pitching, untidy, ragged circle of dancers. What is apparent, is that this is a jolly, social, communal gathering. The dancers zig-zag, talk, jig or skip just as they feel, paying little or no attention to the music. They are much too preoccupied with making themselves agreeable to their neighbours than in learning to dance. To these visitors, it is fun to join the circle and take off their coats, place them, and their handbags, on the ground in the centre of the circle, along with those belonging to the other dancers. They are in ribald mood but dutifully follow their neighbours and try to copy what they see the others are doing. It does not matter how frightful their dancing is, the courteous Spaniards will compliment them, because they are pleased to have them in their midst—they will even praise their rapidity in learning the sardana, for the Catalans consider that it takes years to learn it properly.

What emerges very clearly when witnessing the many circular groups of dancers is that although the outer form of the dance may be communicated to others, the inner meaning is much too subtle to be casually picked up by the visitor and therefore, the dance cannot really be passed on to all and sundry. This seems to me to be inherent in all Spanish dancing and it is in these collective folk-dances that the real quality of the dancing is revealed possibly as in no other type of Spanish dance.

Examples of circle dances are not confined to the east coast. The north possesses one of great interest on account of its antiquity, known as the 'danza prima' which comes from Asturias (pl. 59). It may be remembered that the Asturians lived their own lives behind the mountain ranges while the rest of Spain was dispersing much energy reclaiming their land from the Moors, therefore many vestiges of an ancient civilization may be sought in their dances. The danza prima may be Greek in origin and, like most circle dances, it is of a solemn nature. Boys and girls dance together, there are no rhythmical complications, no leaps, springs, beats or similar strenuous movements that normally distinguish dances from the north. The eighteenth-century writer Jovellanos liked to contrast the serenity of the danza prima with the strong affected 'contortions' of 'modern dances' and observed: 'The slow and ordered movements of this ancient dance are evidence of peaceful and innocent hearts'.

The cori-cori is another Asturian dance of a different type. Alleged to be Celtic in origin, it is an example of a fertility dance, accompanied by bagpipes, tambourines, drums and castanets. In triple time and danced by six girls and one boy, it commences with a ceremonial entrance, the girls incline from the waist, the boy bows. He then skips backwards in a series of 'temps levés'—hop and a jump—on a half turn. Holding branches, the girls advance in file performing one step only—the pas de Basque. First in a lateral direction, then facing inwards and outwards. The beauty of the dance lies in the reiteration of one simple step combined with changing ground patterns.

From the Asturias also comes the vaqueira, with a novel accompaniment of frying pan and tambourine. Asturian too, is the pericote de llanes, winding in a serpentine of figures of eight, completely Celtic in origin but accompanied by castanets. Before leaving the subject of ancient dances, reference should be made in passing to a primitive specimen to be found in the province of Santander. This dance has survived from remote times and is too old for anyone to know when it originated. Dressed in animal skins, and to the accompaniment of ancient horns that make weird sounds (peculiarly like fog horns at sea to modern ears) the dancers go through movements of a warlike nature. This is but one of the many curious old dances to be found in the north. They are real museum pieces, scarcely known outside Spain and well worth recording.

A Celtic flavour is immediately apparent as one approaches the north-western province of Galicia (pl. 61). The form of the dances resembles those from Scotland. The arms are carried at shoulder level, like the horns of a bull, most of the steps are performed on the ball of the foot and the ground pattern is frequently that of a square. Bagpipes, as well as castanets, provide the accompaniment and four or eight dancers perform. Some of the dances are of a very sentimental nature and scallop shells serve to accompany them. These 'coquilles de St. Jacques' refer of course to the patron saint of Spain, St. James.

Bagpipes have existed in Galicia and Asturias for many generations. Outrageous though the idea may seem to many Scots, there is a belief that the Scots got their bagpipes from England; similarly in Spain, many believe that theirs came from Scotland, introduced into the north of Spain by Scottish fishermen who for centuries had been trading with the Spaniards. Like so many other things in Spain, however, this is all very hypothetical.

Other discernible elements in Galician dances are similar to those from Slavonic countries. The variable moods of the music range from a lyric melancholy to gay liveliness which is not unlike those rhythmic variations found in many Russian tunes. These rapid changes from grave to gay influence the dance movements and, moreover, many of the steps in the male dances are identical with those found in Russian dances, as for example when the men squat on their heels as in 'prisiadkas' or leap spiralling into the air, and perform 'cat steps' and 'tours en l'air'. The vigour and violence of male dancing in Galicia is contrasted with the tender, wistful, nostalgic quality found in the girls' dances who sometimes softly accompany themselves by gently scraping together the scallop shells already referred to. The chief attraction of this kind of Spanish dancing lies in the variety of movement and contrast of mood; it may be of a bright, solemn, virile, graceful nature, or completely still, yet full of action at one and the same time. For this reason, Galician dancing has enormous dramatic possibilities, is spectacular by its virtuosity and therefore especially suitable for the theatre.

Antonio was, as far as I know, the first Spanish dance artist to take Galician folk material and attempt to create a complete danced divertissement out of it. When rehearsals started, the Spanish boys were surprised to find that performing these strenuous dances every night made them very stiff. To counteract this stiffness, they were taught basic character barre exercises to warm the muscles—such as those used in other national dancing of a theatrical nature. They found them very beneficial. These dances were never intended to be done night after night, week in, week out, for, in their normal surroundings, they were for high-days and holidays only. It was not so much the actual movements that caused the strain but the prolonged muscular effort required by constant rehearsals and regular performances. There was no more trouble, once the dancers had understood the necessity of preparing their muscles gradually. This is a point that will have to be considered when the Spanish theatre comes into existence and choreographers start adapting this folk material on a wholesale scale!

No less interesting was the reaction of London audiences when they too were first introduced to this novelty. Those who visualized Spanish dancing as nothing more than Andalusians in long-tailed skirts, making a lot of noise with castanets, were dismayed to the point that one member of the audience was heard to remark that he did not know that Spaniards did Polish dancing as well! Yet another indignantly refuted it entirely as not being 'authentic' Spanish dancing. Yet, only the month before, 20,000 Gallegos in Vigo had cheered the same suite—an unlikely thing for them to have done if anything bogus, masquerading as Galician dancing, had been offered them! What is and what is not Spanish dancing is liable to remain a problem among foreign audiences as long as only one facet is administered to them—rather like a medicine labelled 'dose as before'—that is, already known to succeed.

One of the most interesting facets of national dancing in Spain, at least to ballet dancers, is that coming from the Basque country (pl. 60). There is good reason for this, because it is vaguely familiar to them. For generations, Basque steps have been most successfully incorporated into classical ballet technique. In the seventeenth century, it was a Basque who was brought to Paris to, instruct the pupils at the newly-formed Académie de Danse and since that time, the development of ballet technique has owed much to the Basques. This ancient race possesses its own language, believed to be the oldest in the Peninsula. Their dances are equally venerated by age. They have certain points in common with those from other lands as, for instance, when they dance on a tumbler, as also do the Hungarians and other Central European inhabitants. They have their Sword dances, not unlike those performed in Scotland and the Balkans. Finally, the famous 'hobby horse' familiar to all dancers in England, Germany, Austria and Poland.

As a rule, Basque dances are of a concerted nature—sometimes a girl and boy together, at others, all men or all women dancing in a team. In this case, the dances are divided into sections in such a way that individual dancers have a chance of showing off their technical virtuosity. This is of a very high order indeed, particularly amongst the men, who are remarkable for the height they can jump. High leaps into the air, with legs far apart in a wide second position, high kicks, unusual among male dancers, are believed to be a remnant of an ancient fertility rite. Tours en l'air are quite commonplace and the men do them brilliantly. Basque dances sparkle by reason of the most intricate footwork done by both girls and boys, particularly in the rapid beaten steps. It is not surprising that Basque dances lend themselves so successfully for stage purposes.

A prominent feature in Basque dances that is not commonly found in Spanish dancing as a whole, is that the faces of the dancers, when they dance, are quite impassive. This is exactly the reverse in southern Spain, where facial expression or 'the dance of the eyes' is so important. The carriage of the arms is also peculiar to Basque dances in that the hands are kept quietly down by the sides of the body. This carriage of the arms is also characteristic of Irish dancing, for the Irish claim that the 'divil's in the eyes and heels'. Certain tunes are also common to both countries; the ancient Irish melody 'The Little Red Dog' is identical with one used in a Basque dance bearing another title altogether. So far, little has come to light to account for these similarities. It has been suggested that the wrecked Armada off the Irish coast might have exerted some influence, but it seems improbable that Spanish ships were manned exclusively by Basques, or that they were the only survivors! In the musical field one finds Basque tunes cropping up constantly. In Portugal, which in ancient days was joined to what we now call Spain, they dance their national dance, the fandango, to identical Basque tunes, although the steps are totally different from those performed by the Basques to the same melody. A fascinating field of investigation awaits someone here!

The most universally known and probably the most highly esteemed aspect of Spanish dancing abroad is that known as 'Gitano', or Spanish gypsy dancing. It is also the most complex group of all, in a class apart, and for that reason, has been deliberately left until the last. Strictly speaking, Spanish gypsy dancing is another facet of Andalusian regional dancing. Its complexity lies in the fact that at the present moment it is not really known with any degree of certainty where the Spanish gypsies came from before they reached Spain. Some say they came from India, indeed there is a widespread belief that this is so, but those gypsies with whom I worked, absolutely refuted this theory. In their opinion, the English tribes came from India and they based their conclusions on the fact that, when they visited them in Kent, the English gypsies could not speak their language. The Spanish gypsies speak Caló—the English gypsies do not. My Gitano friends thought the English gypsies were related to the Hungarian tribes known as Zingari who, so they said, had migrated from India. According to the gypsies inhabiting Spain today, their people came originally from Egypt and hence the name Gitano. What we should like to know, and cannot find out, is what they brought to Spain in the way of dance material? Of what did their own dances consist, if they had any, and if they had, did they incorporate them with Spanish dances they found in the Peninsula, or merely adopt what they found there and make them their own?

In Andalusia today, the gypsies jealously guard what they have. Dancing to them is a cult so enclosed that it almost amounts to a form of freemasonry. They do not willingly share it with non-gypsies. They claim that Spaniards from other regions can't do it —the Catalans are too cold, the Castilians too serious. As for foreigners, they are totally excluded. Gypsies distinguish between the Andalusian dancing performed by the non-gypsy inhabitants of Andalusia whose basic dances belong to the fandango family, as we have already observed, and their own, but both come under the heading of Andalusian regional dancing. In its own environment, gypsy dancing is hermetically sealed off from the rest of the world.

Taking into consideration that the gypsies entered the Andalusian region so long ago, becoming Spanish in the process, it is strange to find today that these people maintain this 'what I have, I hold' attitude. Such a strong racial feeling must have deep roots indeed, possibly a throwback to the time when the gypsies had such a fierce struggle to survive during the Spanish Inquisition. It might even go further back still, a relic of some ancient religious cult that forbade initiates to divulge their knowledge to the uninitiated.

Whatever the reason, this possessive state of mind prevails and makes it very difficult to obtain real information.

If there is speculation about the origin of the gypsies in Spain, there is just as much about the date of their arrival. Most people, including themselves, seem to think that they began to settle in the Peninsula some time in the fifteenth century. Nomads, they were known for their illiteracy.[2] In 1555, the gypsy origin of the celebrated 'cantaor' Juan de Wrede was doubted, solely on the grounds that he had graduated from Zaragoza University and was a Bachelor of Arts of Valladolid. The duke of Alba, defending him, saw no reason why any relative of a gypsy—even a grandson—should not hold academic titles. In those days, it was so inconceivable, however, that the opposition would not accept it, declaring that these educational qualifications conclusively proved that he was no gypsy, but Asturian, or else a man from some other part of the Peninsula.

Education of a conventional nature may not have existed, but gypsy children learned about the history of their race and the land in which they lived by means of folk-lore handed down from generation to generation. Battles, victories and defeats were recalled in their ballads, events of their daily lives and miracles worked in the lives of the saints were immortalized in their songs, for the Gitanos belong to a pious race—in Spain, they are devout Roman Catholics. St. Sara is their patron saint, and on her name day, tribes coming from various parts of Europe congregate in France to celebrate it together. Their well-known 'cante hondo' or 'deep song' is said to be related to Byzantine liturgical music and this music has been extensively used both in their singing and dancing. 'Deep song' is in the nature of a lament and death is an ever-recurrent theme. The art of the Gitanos stems from the outpouring of deep racial feeling and accumulated suffering, born of the persecution of their race in the past. The daily prayer of the Gitano is for 'health and liberty' and no more fitting symbol could be found for their dancing. Their strength is the outcome of a healthy determination to survive, and reflects the religious dignity of their daily lives. The 'duende' or spirit expressed in their dances is the outward expression of an inner striving for freedom.

[2]Duke of Alba: *Discursos*; private archives.

'Duende' cannot be translated into English. It is closely related to the Welsh 'hwll' and is never far absent from Gitano dances when performed in their natural surroundings. When the Gitanos are possessed by this 'duende' they appear to be in a state of trance. A theatre is not necessary to enter this spiritual kingdom. A gypsy mother may pause in the midst of her daily chores to lose herself in a fragment of song or dance. The rest of the family will stop whatever they are doing to gather round to watch, appraise and enter into this brief moment of communion with her. They may even actively participate with her, thus sharing a fugitive escape from the commonplace things of life. There is an air of ritual about the proceedings and, like most intimate things in life, may not be shared with everybody. By its nature, it can only be restricted to those who understand and feel in the same way. Poignancy is added to the performance by the special deference paid to the person possessed, by the other members of the tribe, as though they were taking part in family prayers. Sober and solemn, the essence of Gitano dancing in its proper surroundings is religious or something very akin to it.

If only for this reason, it is difficult to see how this type of dance can be adequately translated into theatrical terms to entertain the crowd for, after all, the primary function of the theatre is surely to entertain? Once weaned away from the caves and encampments of Andalusia, Gitano dancing is forced to undergo radical changes to a degree far in excess of any other less intimate kind of Spanish regional dance. Because of its popularity abroad, Spanish gypsy dancing is being increasingly exploited commercially. So much so that at times it has already reached such a point as to be almost unrecognizable. Among audiences it has become a mania and one reason for this is that people are no longer content just to watch, they want to do it. This is all to the good, provided that these 'fans', in their zeal, do not force and exaggerate the physical aspect at the expense of the emotional content of this highly sensitive and subtle form of dance expression. These lovers of flamenco form a large part of the new international audiences who cannot see too much of it, but they tend to make excessive demands upon the genuine artists who, complying, also force themselves into such a state of muscular strain and nervous exhaustion that any message they set out to give is overpowered by self-conscious effort! It would appear that there are three principal factors that contribute to the changes that are at present taking place in theatrical Gitano dancing commonly called flamenco. Firstly, too frequent repetition of the same dances to please the rapacious appetites of the foreign 'flamencomaniacs'. Secondly, the extreme stylization that has been found necessary to meet the needs of unfamiliar surroundings such as large theatres or open-air stadiums. Lastly, and perhaps the most important one of all, since the artists themselves are responsible for it, is the exaggerated mimicry to simulate the anguish that so many flamenco dancers are addicted to express these days. This can never replace the serene gravity that is the quintessence of the original. A process of synthesis is slowly distorting the original shape of this most intimate, hierarchic and individualistic form of dancing. It has come to be generally known as 'flamenco dancing', and is in reality a distorted theatricalized version of Andalusian regional dancing. Practised more and more by non-gypsies, it is in danger of losing the racial symbolism that distinguishes it from all the other regional dances of Spain.

The world-wide popularity of Flamenco dancing is a curious phenomenon of post-war years. Before the Second World War, a 'cuadro flamenco' at the London Coliseum made little or no impact upon the English audiences. After the bleakness of war-time, however, public taste changed. As one after the other, Spanish dance companies came to enchant them, British audiences accorded them an uncommonly warm reception. It may have been the life, colour and movement that helped to lift the English out of the lethargy caused by wartime regimentation—added to the intrinsic value of the fine dancing that was then to be seen. These Spanish groups were small and their performances of an intimate kind, and this in itself made an instant appeal to the Anglo-Saxons, thus creating a public demand for Spanish dancing in sophisticated theatres.

Gone are those days. So many people, at least in England, tend to confuse Spanish with flamenco dancing to such a degree that to the man in the street, flamenco is the only Spanish dancing he recognizes; it means furiously flashing eyes, taut muscles, contorted expressions of the face, plenty of heel-tapping and finger-snapping and the more noise made, the better people like it. This association of ideas is of relatively recent date and can be identified with the sincere admiration that has grown almost into a passion for this form of dancing. Flamencomania has become a natural consequence of this passion. But it has no roots in Spain. Indeed it puzzles many Spaniards who wonder how it has come to thrive so healthily among foreigners in their coffee-bars, cabarets, cinemas and theatres? Spanish dancers are not slow to realize the material benefits accruing from this mania and adopt more and more cosmopolitan gimmicks in order to please this new international public. If exaggeration brings applause, they exaggerate, and it follows from this that the foreign fans copy them when they try to master the intricacies of flamenco. What is perhaps the most racial and formal of all Spanish dancing is in the guise of flamenco slowly becoming standardized and there are signs that many erstwhile admirers are now finding it a bore for this reason. This is probably only a phase and will pass, but if it does not, Spanish gypsy dancing will become less and less Andalusian and correspondingly more commercially successful than ever. Jazz flamenco has already come and gone, who knows what will follow?

It might have been hoped that the theatre could have preserved all that is best in Andalusian gypsy dancing, but it seems to be little more than an outlet for extrovert gypsies, and others, to show their wares. There is more scope abroad than at home for this sort of exhibitionism and obviously it is more lucrative than dealing in horses, telling fortunes or peddling tourist knick-knacks. What the dancers are in danger of forgetting in the first flush of their enormous success is, that the international theatre can never replace the region as a focal point of genuine Gitano 'duende'—or inspiration—nor are foreign flamencomaniacs capable of replacing the discerning audiences of their own people. Intimacy is necessary in the first place, to induce that state of grace and essential stillness that begets the 'duende'. That kind of dancing known as flamenco is departing from the controls placed upon it by the gypsies themselves and assuming the accent of the alien land, wherever it may be, finally to settle and there to gell.

Flamenco, of course, does not mean Spanish in the first place—even when applied to dancing—it means Fleming, Flemish, or merely non-Spanish. The use of the word in common parlance dates from the time when there was a good deal of Flemish influence about in Spain. Charles I of Spain was born in Ghent and was surrounded by Flemish nobles when he was called to the throne and they accompanied him to Spain. There were close commercial ties between Seville and Antwerp in the sixteenth century and these brought many Flemish settlers to Spain. The Spanish soldiers of the army of occupation were themselves known as 'Flamencos'. When these Spanish troops returned to Spain from Flanders they brought with them many Flemish nationals who, naturally, were known as 'Flamencos' and their arrival happened to coincide with that of large numbers of gypsies settling in the Peninsula. Thus, in the minds of Spaniards, flamenco was a collective term applied to those people in their midst of non-Spanish origin. Flamenco therefore would appear to be quite a suitable name for this curious mixture of dancing that recognizes no territorial boundary and is now rampant throughout the world.

Today, there is no other type of Spanish dancing that can vie with it for filling the theatre. At times it has been known to reduce audiences to a state bordering on hysteria. Yet, in spite of the deep emotional feelings it engenders among dancers and public alike, it does not seem to have inspired anybody to create any original flamenco choreography. The set dances like polos, zorongos, gitanos and tiranas appear to satisfy everybody. It might have been thought that, now that it is so firmly established in the new medium of the theatre, some Gitano choreographer might have emerged. Flamenco has been on the stage long enough for some choreographic seeds to have sprouted. That this has not happened may mean that the gypsies have no inherent gift for choreography. In Spain, they have not had much opportunity of proving their worth in this direction, since there has never been a theatre devoted to gypsy lore—such as there was in Russia before the revolution.

It may be surmised that *baile nacional* began to take the shape that we see today in the sixteenth century, as visual, literary and musical evidence gradually became available. Prior to that period, as was observed in the early chapters of this book, conclusions were reached mainly through speculation. It may be remembered that the first Spanish document about which we can be sure, dates from the fifteenth century. Then, after the establishment of the court of the Catholic kings, and only then, did new dance creations and innovations become apparent. Provençal influences were strong among the troubadours in the thirteenth century and these permeated the north of the Peninsula, while Arab influence was all-powerful in the south. There was a dual movement from north to south and from south to north. The northern dances were often of an archaic nature while those from the south were the products of the Arabs, who were innovators. Throughout the tempestuous times of the Reconquest, a mixture of races of diverse origin had to be moved to repopulate the country. Many were the descendants of the Visigoths, Moriscos and Mozarabes, who had conserved the ancient dance forms and these were the people who travelled south, east and west to occupy the new-found territories. This movement of the people in the process of repopulation was a most important factor in the development of the dances of the period. It implied slow evolution, finding another level, more evolution and as this process never stopped, while so many people of diverse origin kept moving about the country over a long period of time, the dances of old were added to by newer and newer creations. There can be no doubt that the different dance-forms were directly related to the exploits of a historical nature that were then taking place. Spanish dancing became solidified as a result of the unification of the country and made still more rapid strides after the sixteenth century, constantly developing through the centuries into what we now see.

Enough has been said about Spanish national dancing to indicate why there is such immense variety in the steps, rhythmic pattern, and design of *baile nacional*. Only a fraction of this material has been uncovered and that is what is seen in the theatre today. A rich storehouse awaits anybody who has the time, energy and enthusiasm to unearth its treasures. Much is still hidden away and covers too wide a field of unrelated knowledge for dancers or choreographers to sift, alone and unaided. Expert help is needed to sort it out and one would imagine that the right people to give that required assistance would be experienced anthropologists, historians and musicologists.

Further research would be useful to ascertain, for example, what influence colonial expansion had upon Spanish dancing. It has been suggested that the sarabande and chaconne had a very shady past but, beyond a hint that this was related to the fact that these dances were imported from the colonies, the reason why remains a mystery. Much also needs to be done to clarify the musical situation. Liturgical music is said to have influenced the musical form of that belonging to the Jewish and Moorish inhabitants of Spain and it may be assumed that early Spanish dance form fell under similar influences. Dance form closely follows the same lines as musical form. As for the most intriguing topic of Spanish Gitano dancing, many questions need answering. An adequate survey of the symbolism underlying Spanish gypsy art can hardly begin, until there is some degree of certainty concerning where the Spanish gypsy tribes originated in the first place.

So much for the content of dance material in *baile nacional* and the need for more detailed investigation. The attitude of cosmopolitan audiences towards it and the influence they are exerting has been mentioned, but what of the Spanish public? There are some who deplore the tendency to pander to foreign taste by refining the old folk dances just to please the box offices of the world. There are quite as many however, who see in this trend great balletic possibilities in the future. They are at a loss to understand why a Spanish ballet company does not already exist. The writers, painters and composers of Spanish nationality abound in the homeland—both classical and modern—and they are all ready for their creations to be used. All the necessary adjuncts for a national ballet are there. What then, is everybody waiting for? The answer is quite simple— all that is needed is a base, to harness all these resources, in the form of a subsidized theatre.

Epilogue

PLANS ARE now under way to found a national theatre in Madrid, specializing in the production of opera and ballet. By the munificence of the late Juan March, a sum of money was left to the state for this purpose. The theatre will not be built on the site of the old Royal Opera House but in the modern part of the capital.

The old Real is now used as a headquarters for the nationally-subsidized orchestras. The stage has been transformed into a concert platform and used for concerts of all kinds. Following its chequered career, an attempt was made in this year of grace 1969, to set it on fire during the Eurovision contests. This was alleged to be an effort to sabotage the competition.

As for the proposed new theatre, nobody yet knows what form it will take. A competition has been held for designs which have already been submitted. If, as seems possible, the heir to the Spanish throne is crowned, who knows, the company may be again named 'royal' and 'going to the ballet' may be revived as a social custom. The 'Royal Spanish Ballet' might come once more to London to charm the audiences, as did its predecessor of the same name in the last century at the old Alhambra.

The important point is that this theatre is no longer the distant dream that it has been for so long. Be it royal or national, within the space of a few years the Spanish Ballet is to be ensconced in a permanent theatre in the metropolis. An event of the utmost importance to the future Dancing Spaniards!

There may be some cynics who want to know who cares anyway whether or not there is an opera house in Madrid? Apparently the authorities care. Then there are the legions of Spanish dancers; perhaps they care more than anybody else, for they are anxiously awaiting its establishment. Here, I should point out that when referring to Spanish dancers, I have in mind dancers from Spain and not, unless otherwise stated, professional dancers from other lands who perform Spanish dances. It is the Dancing Spaniards who long for the day when, thanks to state support, they will be provided with stable conditions under which to study and work and, finally, attain a prestige hitherto denied them. The fact that their company is to receive official blessing in the form of a national subsidy may do much, they feel, to remove the old social stigma attached to 'dancing in the theatre'.

What provision will be made for the Spanish dancers once the theatre, complete with studios and rehearsal rooms, is inaugurated? Earlier on it was observed that a physical theatre was not enough in itself, unless a company existed inside to bring it to life. It was also stated that a nucleus of Spanish dancers already exists having gained theatrical experience by dancing in privately owned companies. A useful beginning to any company indeed, but this nucleus does not constitute a company. Much more has to be done; an artistic policy has to be produced, an orchestra also will be indispensable and, last but by no means least, a strong supporting group of dancers will be necessary. A *corps de ballet* will have to be built up and maintained to provide an annual intake of uniformly strong and well-trained dancers. An adequate teaching department will be needed to train them.

Recently an interesting development has taken place. Mariemma has been appointed to teach dancing of the Bolero school, regional dances and 'escola flamenca' at the Royal School of Dramatic Art. She is also scheduled to give lessons in stylization and choreography. This sounds as though a complete Spanish school of theatre is in the process of formation. It is unusual to see 'flamenco' referred to as 'flamenco school' and implies that already a systematic method of teaching has been evolved to teach this subject. Since they have gone so far it may be hoped that soon the most complete discipline for the theatre, known at present in the form of classical ballet technique, will also be considered by the Spanish authorities of sufficient importance to be included in the course. Ultimately, to round off the teaching curriculum supplementary subjects such as character dancing, mime, *pas de deux*, dance history and music classes will bring the teaching programme in line with national instructional establishments elsewhere. For despite their inherited dancing talent, what the Dancing Spaniards of the future do with this, will depend to a large extent upon their artistic formation which, in turn, will be the outcome of the training they have received.

Only after they are adequately equipped theatrically, will the young Spanish dancers be in a position to reforge the broken link that arrested further development of Spanish Ballet after the eighteenth century. Only when they have a working knowledge of stage-craft will budding choreographers have any chance of showing their paces in the realm of Spanish choreography. Once these requirements are met, this modern theatre could well become a forcing ground for the new impulse in ballet that the world is waiting for.

History has a strange way of repeating itself and, as we have seen, there have been in the past periods of slumber. Ballet in Spain has been dormant for some time but the moment of reawakening appears to be at hand. The Dancing Spaniards, conscious of what is happening, are revelling in pleasant anticipation, all too aware that it will be against their long and glorious dance tradition that future balletic achievements in Spain will be assessed. Their own theatre will be not only their hope but also their challenge.

MADRID, LISBON 1962–70

Appendix A

DANCE TUNES TAKEN FROM *LAS CANTIGAS DE ALFONSO EL SABIO* BY JULIAN RIBERA

13 Solea gitano or Playera—apparently Canto Hondo.
23 Similar to a present-day jota.
29 Habanera.
30 Similar to modern Peteneras.
121 A paso doble for the lute.
206 A waltz.
209 Sevillanas 'floreadas'.
230 A popular dance tune.
290 A popular melody from Asturias.
291 A theme that has remained in the Jota Aragonesa.
304 Many tunes such as this are to be found in collections of troubadour music.
313 Andalusian Soleares—the theme of this song was widespread in Spain in medieval and modern times. This theme is Andalusian but was popular in other songs to be found in the centre and north of Spain.
318 Very like the Soleares gitanos of Andalusia.

Appendix B

NOTATION FOR 'FILLES A MARIER'

NOTE: s—simple (or single)
       d—double
       r—reprise
       R—Reverence
       b—branle

For comparison, two versions of 'Filles a Marier', one from Cervera (Spain *c.* 1496), the other from Salisbury (England *c.* 1497). In modern notation.

CERVERA SS. ss. ddd. ss. rrr. b.
         ss.   d. ss. rrr. b.
         ss. ddd. ss. rrr. b.
         ss.   d. ss. rrr. b.

SALISBURY SS. ss. ddd.   rrr. b.
           ss.   d. ss. rrr. b.
           ss. ddd. ss. rrr. b.
           ss.   d.   rrr. b.

Although the two versions do not agree absolutely, they clearly adhere to the strict French rules in basse danse.
(a) Singles must always be in pairs.
(b) Doubles and reprises must always be uneven—one, three or five.
(b) Every measure (or section) must begin SS and end R.B.

The Spanish manuscript *Orleans* is peculiar in suggesting backward movements as well as forward on the singles. Reprises are always back of course.

CERVERA *Orleans*
         R.b. ss. (back)   ddd. rrr. b.
              ss. (forward) d. rrr. b.
              ss. (back)   ddd. rrr. b.
              ss. (back)   d. rrr. b.
              ss. (forward)

(the final ss. would count as a reverence)

Bibliography

ALBA, Duke of, *Discursos*.
ALEMAN, Mateo, *Guzman de Alfarache* (1599).
ALTAMIRA, Rafael, *Manuel de Historia de España* (Buenos Aires 1946).
AMADES, J. y F. Pujol, *Diccionario de la Dansa* (Barcelona).
ANGLES, Higinio, *Diccionario de la Musica* (Barcelona 1954). *La Musica en la Corte de los Reyes Catolicos* (Madrid 1941).
ANTUNA, M., *La Corte Literaria de Alhaguen de Cordoba* (San Lorenzo de Escorial 1929).
Archives Historicos de Toledo, Leg. 2, Fol. 95, Ano 1631 (Biblioteca Nacional, Madrid).
d'AULNOY, La Comtesse, *Lady's Travels in Spain* (London 1708).

BARBIERE, Francisco Asenjo, *Cancionero de los Siglos XV y XVI* (Madrid 1890). *El Teatro Real y el Teatro de la Zarzuela* (Madrid 1877).
BECKFORD, William, *Spanish Journal* (London 1954).
BENAVENTE, Quinones de, *Entremeses* (Zaragoza 1945).
BENOIS, Alexandre, *Reminiscences of the Russian Ballet* (London 1941).
BON, Stella, *Les Grands Courants de la Danse* (Paris 1954).
BONALD, Caballero, *El Baile Andaluz* (Barcelona 1957).
BUSTAMENTE, Perez C., *Compendio de Historia de España* (Madrid 1952).

CAHUSAC, de, *La Danse Ancienne et Moderne* (The Hague 1754).
CALDERON, Estebanez, *Escenas Andaluzas* (Madrid 1833).
CALDERON, Juan Rodrigo Jacinto, *Bolerologia* (Philadelphia 1807).
CALDERON DE LA BARCA, *Autos Sacramentales* (Madrid 1942).
CAPMANY, Aureli, *La Dansa a Catalunya* (Barcelona 1930).
CAROSO, Fabritio, *Il Balerino* (Venice 1581). *Nobilita di Dame* (Venice 1605).
CERVANTES, Miguel de, *Don Quixote de la Mancha* (Madrid 1941). *Entremeses* (Madrid 1952).
COCK, Enrique, *Relacion de Felipe II* (Madrid 1876).
COTARELI Y MORI, *Coleccion de Loas, Bailes, Jacaras y Mojigangas desde Fines Siglo XVI a Mediodias del XVIII* (Madrid 1911). *Historia de la Zarzuela* (Madrid 1934). *Origenes y Establecimiento de la Opera en España hasta 1800* (Madrid 1917).

Bibliography

COTARELO Y VALEDOR, *Historia Critica y Documentada de la Vida de Alfonso III el Magno* (Madrid 1933).

COURNAND, Gilberte (Coll. and ed. by), *Press Extracts on* La Argentina (Paris 1928–36).

COVARRUBIAS, *Tesoro de la Lengua Castellana* (1611).

CRUZ, Ramon de la, *La Junta de los Payos (1761)* (Madrid 1941).

DELEITE Y PINUELA, J., *El Origen y Apogée del Genero Chico en España* (Madrid 1947). *El Rey se divierte* (Madrid 1935). *Tambien se divierte el Pueblo* (Madrid 1944).

DON PRESCISO (J. A. de Iza Zamacola y Ozerian), *Elementos de la Ciencia Contradanzaria* (Madrid 1796).

DOZY, R., *Histoire des Musulmans d'Espagne jusqu'à la Conquête d'Andalousie (711–1110)* (Leyden 1932).

ELLIS, Havelock, *The Soul of Spain* (New York 1920).

ESQUIVEL DE NAVARRO, *Discursos sobre el Arte del Danzado* (Seville 1642).

FARMER, Henry, *History of Arabian Music* (London 1929).

FERNANDEZ Y GONZALEZ, *Estudio Social y Politico de los Mudejares en Castilla* (Madrid 1866).

FERRIO Y BOXERAUS, *Explicaciones de la Corografia* (Malaga 1745).

FEUILLET, R. A., 'Choréographie' ou l'Art de décrire la Danse (Paris 1701).

GARCIA, Gomez E., *Cinco Poetas Musulmanes* (Madrid 1944). *Poemas Arabigoandaluces* (España-Calpe).

GAUTIER, Théophile, *Wanderings in Spain* (London 1853).

GINES, Perez de Hita, *Las Guerras Civiles de Granada (1595)*.

GONZALEZ Palencia, *Historia de la España Musulmana* (Barcelona 1932).

GRAMMONT, Duc de, *Diario*.

HERRERO, Bernabe, *Cante, Baile y Música Española* (Madrid 1957).

ISIDORE, St, of Seville, *Etymologia* (Madrid 1951).

JAQUE, Ivan Antonio, *Libro de danzar de D. de Rojas Panteja* (Mss. National Library, Madrid).

JOVELLANOS, *Espectaculos Publicos y su Origen en España* (Granada 1820).

LAUZE, F. de, *Apologie de la Danse* (Paris 1623).

LEVINSON, A., *Marie Taglioni* (trans. C. Beaumont) (London 1930).

LEVI-PROVENÇAL, *Alphonse VI et la Prise de Tolède* (Madrid 1931). *España Musulmana* (Madrid 1930).

LOPE DE VEGA, *Obras Completas* (Madrid 1944).

MAGRI, G., *Trattate Prattico di Balle* (1788).

MARCAIS, Georges, *Le Monde Orientale de 395–1081* (Paris 1936).

MARIANO, Padre, *Libro de los Espectaculos* (sixteenth century).

MARMOL, *Rebelión de los Moriscos* (1600).

Bibliography

MARRERO, Vincente, *El Enigma de España en la Danza Española* (Madrid 1959).
MATOS, Garcia G., *Viejas Canciones y Melodias en la Musica Popular* (Barcelona 1958).
MAURA, Gamazo G., *Rincones de la Historia* (Madrid 1941).
MENENDEZ, Pidal, *Historia de la España* (Madrid 1940).
MICHAUT, Pierre, *Danse Espagnole* (Paris 1949).
MINQUET Y YROT, *El Noble Arte de Danzar* (Madrid 1758).
MITJANA, Rafael, *La Mucique en Espagne* (Paris 1920).
MUÑOZ, Mathilde, *Historia del Teatro Real, Madrid* (Madrid 1946).

NAVARRETE Y RIBERA, *Flor de Sainete* (1690).
NEGRI, Cesare, *Nueve Invenzioni di Balli* (Milan 1604).
NOVERRE, *Lettres sur la Danse et sur les Ballets* (Stuttgart 1760).

PÉCOUR ET FEUILLET, *Recueil de Danses* (Paris 1709).
PEDRELL, Felipe, *Cancionero Musical Popular Español* (Barcelona 1948).
PELLICER, Casiano, *La Comedia en España* (Madrid 1804).
PEREZ, Pujol, *Historia de las Instituciones Sociales de la España Goda* (Valencia 1896).
PERUGINI, Mark, *The Art of the Ballet* (London 1915).
PRIETO, Vives A., *Formación del Reino de Granada* (Madrid 1929). *Los Reyes de Taifas* (Madrid 1925).

QUEROL, Miguel, *La Música de las Obras de Cervantes* (Barcelona 1948).
QUEVEDO, *Obras Completas* (Madrid 1945).
RAMEAU, *Le Maître à danser* (Paris 1725).
Relaciones Historicas de los Siglos XVI y XVII (Madrid 1896).
RIBERA, J., *La Musica de las Cantigas* (Madrid 1922).
RIBERA Y TARRAGA, *La Música Andaluza Medaeval en las Canciones de los Troveres* (Madrid 1929). *La Música de la Jota Aragonesa* (Madrid 1928).
RIEGO, Fernando del, *Danzas Populares Gallegas* (Buenos Aires 1950).
RIOS, Amador de los, *Historia Social, Literaria y Politica de los Judios en España* (Madrid 1951).
ROJAS, Fray Fernandez de, *Crotalogia* (Madrid 1792).
RUBIO Y BALGUER, *Vida Española en la Época Gotica* (Barcelona 1943).

SACHS, Curt, *Histoire de la Danse* (Paris 1938).
SALAZAR, Adolfo, *La Musica en España* (Buenos Aires 1953). *La Musica en la Sociedad Europea* (Mexico 1944). *Sinfonia y Ballet* (Madrid 1929).
SALAZAR, Eugenio (born 1530), *Cartas*.
SANCHEZ, Albornez, *Estampes de la Vida en Leon durante el Siglo X.* (Madrid 1926).
SCHNEIDER, Marius, *La Danza de Espadas y la Tarantela* (Barcelona 1948).
SIMONET, F. S., *Sacada de los Autores Arabigos* (Granada 1827).
STARKIE, Walter, *Don Gypsy* (London 1936). *In Sara's Tents* (London 1953).
STRABO, *Geografía* (Madrid 1737).
SUBIRA, José, *Historia de la Musica* (Barcelona 1947). *Historia y Anecdotas del Teatro Real* (Madrid 1949). *La Tonadilla Escénica* (Madrid 1928).

Bibliography

TABANERA, Manuel, *Tesoro de Folklore Español.*
TERRELLAS, Albert, *Lola Montes, la Amada del Rey,—poeta* (Barcelona 1944).
TORRES, Manuel, *El Estado Visigodo*

VAILLAT, Leandre, *La Taglioni* (Paris 1942).
VALLADOR, F., *Apuntes para la Historia de la Musica en Granada* (Granada 1922).
VILLANUEVA, *Viaje Literária a las Iglesias de España* (Valencia 1821).
VUILLIER, Gaston, *La Danse* (Paris 1895).

WEAVER, John, *An Essay towards a History of Dancing* (London 1712).
WOOD, Melusine, *Advanced Historical Dances* (London 1960). *English Country Dance prior to the seventeenth century.*

ZAZO, *Historia del Real* (Madrid 1956).
ZAZO, Antonio Velasco, *La Seguidilla* (Madrid 1918).

Acknowledgements

First, I am indebted to Eduardo de Aranda of the Spanish Embassy, Caracas and his wife Isabel, for their faith in this work and never failing help and encouragement over a period of many years.

I should also like to gratefully acknowledge the inestimable value of the assistance given to me by Dr Ernesto de la Orden, Spanish Ambassador in Nicaragua, who kindly read the original rough draft and encouraged me to publish the book. Thanks are also due to his successor Don Eduardo Toda, Cultural Counsellor Spanish Embassy, London, for reading the final manuscript and kindly informing the Ministerio de Informacion y Turismo of its existence, culminating in practical aid which has hastened along publication.

No words can adequately express my profound gratitude to His Excellency the Spanish Ambassador in Ankara Don Emilio Garcia Gomez and his wife Maria Luisa, whose interest in my work threw wide open all the doors at the Biblioteca Nacional, Madrid and so expedited what otherwise might have been an onerously lengthy task.

My grateful thanks are due to the Director of the Biblioteca Nacional, Madrid—Don Guillermo Guastavine and his splendid staff for their courteous attention to my many problems.

I am indebted to Frances Bell Macdonald for all her patience and perseverance in reading and correcting the rough drafts. To Cecily Grant for the many weary hours she spent typing and re-typing the first manuscript. To Margaret Thain, Librarian at the Spanish Institute, London, who tirelessly hunted up sources of information for me and made them readily available.

Acknowledgements

I am grateful to Nalda Murilooh for looking over printer's proofs and for her many helpful suggestions.

I should like to express my deep appreciation to Luis Marques and his wife Susan Lowndes for their great kindness in reading and editing the final typescript.

To my old friend Catherine Hutter go my warmest thanks for her helpful suggestions regarding the publication of this book, particularly with reference to the United States.

Finally a deep debt of gratitude to Melusine Wood who fostered in me an interest in dance research and taught me all I know about dance history.

Index

Index